G000320351

Psychodynamic approaches
to sexual problems

*Psychodynamic approaches
to sexual problems*

Brian Daines and Angelina Perrett

Open University Press
Buckingham · Philadelphia

Open University Press
Celtic Court
22 Ballmoor
Buckingham
MK18 1XW

e-mail: enquiries@openup.co.uk
world wide web: http://www.openup.co.uk

and

325 Chestnut Street
Philadelphia, PA 19106, USA

First Published 2000

Copyright © Brian Daines and Angelina Perrett 2000

All rights reserved. Except for the quotation of short passages for the purpose of criticism and review, no part of this publication may be reproduced, stored in a retrieval system, or transmitted, in any form or by any means, electronic, mechanical, photocopying, recording or otherwise, without the prior written permission of the publisher or a licence from the Copyright Licensing Agency Limited. Details of such licences (for reprographic reproduction) may be obtained from the Copyright Licensing Agency Ltd of 90 Tottenham Court Road, London, W1P 9HE.

ISBN   0 335 20159 8 (pb)   0 335 20160 1 (hb)

A catalogue record of this book is available from the British Library

Library of Congress Cataloging-in-Publication Data
Daines, Brian.
   Psychodynamic approaches to sexual problems/Brian Daines and Angelina Perrett.
       p.   cm.
   Includes bibliographical references and index.
   ISBN 0-335-20160-1 (hardcover). – ISBN 0-335-20159-8 (pbk.)
   1. Psychosexual disorders–Treatment.   2. Sex therapy.
3. Psychodynamic psychotherapy.   I. Perrett, Angelina, 1960– .
II. Title.
RC557.D35 2000
616.85′830651–dc21   99–39401
                                                                    CIP

Copy-edited and typeset by The Running Head Limited,
www.therunninghead.com
Printed in Great Britain by St Edmundsbury Press Ltd,
Bury St Edmunds, Suffolk

For Joan and Kevin

Contents

List of figures

List of tables

Acknowledgements

While writing this book we have received support and encouragement from many friends and colleagues. In particular we would like to thank the staff of the Porterbrook Clinic for their help, Anita Coan for her assistance with the case histories, and Pam Johnson for her secretarial support. We would also like to thank Michael Jacobs, who encouraged us to write this book and has given valuable editorial advice and support.

Introduction

This book explores the application of psychodynamic theories and techniques to clients in counselling or psychotherapy who have sexual difficulties. However, it is not aimed only at the counsellor or psychotherapist who works entirely in a psychodynamic way. The ideas discussed are also relevant to those who use an integrative approach incorporating psychodynamic ideas and interventions, as well as practitioners who wish to increase their psychodynamic understanding and insights. It provides useful knowledge, for example, for those needing to assess whether a referral to someone using a psychodynamic approach would be appropriate.

Looking back at the way that sexual problems have been approached psychologically reveals a period, starting from Freud and lasting until the emergence of behavioural methods of treating sexual problems in the 1970s, which was dominated by psychoanalysis. Surprisingly, though, psychoanalysts have given little attention specifically to the commonly occurring sexual difficulties, and as a result, within psychoanalysis little of substance has been added to Freud's understanding. It was the work of two physiologists, Masters and Johnson (1966, 1970) that was to revolutionize the treatment of such difficulties both in Britain and the United States from the mid-1970s onwards. The background to their work is to be found within sexology rather than psychotherapy or psychoanalysis.

Belliveau and Richter's (1971) authorized account of Masters and Johnson's work lists only one psychologically minded antecedent, Freud (1905), among the five that they identify. The others are a physician, Ellis (1929, 1936, 1952, 1954), gynaecologists Van der Velde (1930) and Dickinson (1933; Dickinson and Pierson 1925), and a zoologist, Kinsey (Kinsey *et al.* 1948, 1953). The discipline of sexology has continued, particularly in the United States, as an interdisciplinary science involving a wide range of professionals including sociologists, anthropologists, biologist, lawyers and educators, as well as medical doctors and psychologists. Although the origin of the comprehensive application of cognitive and behavioural techniques to sexual problems is commonly traced back to Masters and Johnson's work, their approach is not identified by them in this way.

Thus Bancroft (1997) considers that the original descriptions of their work conveyed, by default, a predominantly behavioural model, but that their subsequent writing reveals that there was much more than this to their treatment. In Britain, the work of Dicks (1967) was very influential in the 1960s in establishing a strong psychodynamic emphasis in couples work, and since then many practitioners have integrated Masters and Johnson's sensate focus techniques into such an approach. More recently influences on sex therapy from family therapy have been evident, in particular the importance of systems approaches (e.g. Crowe 1985; Crowe and Ridley 1990; Bubenzer and West 1993).

In this process the direct application of psychodynamic ideas and techniques to sexual difficulties has tended to be sidelined. As we have noted, historically psychoanalysts have shown great interest in sexual material, but little in the common presenting problems. This has resulted in an interest in sexual psychopathology in terms of paraphilias, but little has been written about the commonly presenting sexual difficulties (Meltzer 1973; Fogel and Myers 1991). In addition to the effect of such historical factors, the assumption tends to be made that a psychodynamic approach to sexual difficulties is less cost-effective than the alternatives, in particular than those based on physical and behavioural interventions. A scepticism about the validity of traditional psychoanalytic understandings in this area, together with a view that using psychoanalysis to treat sexual problems is like taking a sledgehammer to a walnut, has tended to prejudice the exploration and use of more modern analytic and psychodynamic understandings. Additionally there has been a charisma surrounding Masters and Johnson's work and the treatment methods associated with it that has made it difficult for people to consider alternatives dispassionately.

It is also unfortunate that there has been no research in this area to establish whether or not the assumptions made about psychodynamic therapy in relation to sexual problems are true. One reason for this is the comparative ease with which the effectiveness of cognitive-behavioural – as opposed to analytic and psychodynamic – psychotherapies can be investigated and researched: the aims, methods and outcome measures of the former can be more easily defined and quantified. All this created a background against which most therapists working psycho-therapeutically with erectile dysfunction became more inter-ested in exploring cognitive-behavioural psychotherapies when encountering a sexual presenting problem.

By contrast, analytic and psychodynamic psychotherapies have been perceived as longer term and less cost-effective, and as more difficult to integrate with allied helping techniques, such as educational and medical interventions. The political and cultural climate of the last twenty years, with its emphasis on immediate gratification, has also been influential. The result has often not been conducive to more reflective approaches, which tend to be more associated with the culture of the 1960s and 1970s.

Another important development that has directly affected the field of psychosexual work has been the massive input of resources in the 1990s into the area of male erectile problems. This has led to the development of oral preparations, injections, mechanical devices, and the establishment of male erectile dys-function clinics often using an exclusively medical approach to the difficulties.

In part this has been a response to the fact that a predomi-nantly organic basis can be established for many cases of erectile dysfunction. This has fuelled ideas of quick-fix solutions to diffi-culties that are in reality embedded in quite complex psycho-logical and relational settings. This in turn threatens to increase the polarization of views about the kinds of therapeutic interven-tions that are most effective in such cases. Riley (1998) points out the tendency for practitioners to focus selectively on particular components of a sexual problem, according to training and ex-perience. It is important to adopt a broader approach that takes into account the psychosocial, physiological and psychological aspects of the problem, both in the client and in the partner (if there is one). There is still a lack of knowledge about the way that the differing component parts of human sexual function interact and how the impact of each can vary between individuals. It is therefore important to recognize that mechanical and pharmacological treatments that restore physiological function do nothing to address intrapsychic or relationship issues. In some cases the restoration of physiological function brings tensions to a head by changing the psychological equilibrium within the relationship (see Levine 1992; Riley 1998; Segraves and Segraves 1998).

The rush to idealize such treatments is contra-indicated by the evidence from research studies; these reveal high dropout rates, which are 40 to 60 per cent higher than when drugs alone are used (Althof *et al.* 1991; Godschalk *et al.* 1996). This suggests that, whatever the origins of some of these difficulties, people need a multifaceted approach. Without appropriate psychological intervention, the indications are that any lasting positive benefits will not be sustained. Furthermore, the clinician who is unskilled in understanding relationship dynamics may well unwittingly precipitate a crisis in the relationship by ignoring the partner of a man with erectile problems and the dynamics of the relationship (Segraves and Segraves 1998). As Althof and Turner (1992) have noted, many men have hoped that the cavernosal self-injection would improve their marriage, although this seldom occurs. The gender differences in perception of these difficulties is also an important aspect that is often neglected when sexual problems are treated in isolation from the relationships in which these problems occur. Many men will identify the sexual problem as the sole difficulty, yet interviewing partners reveals that they are also concerned with other issues, such as lack of communication, lack of intimacy, power struggles, child-care issues, and other matters that they identify as creating discontent.

The role of sexual problems in regulating intimacy and containing emotional problems is well documented (Leiblum and Rosen 1992; Levine 1992; LoPiccolo 1992). The case for revisiting sexual problems from a psychodynamic perspective is made by Scharff and Scharff (1991: x), who state that any sexual difficulty 'obviously affects marriage in the initiation and maintenance phases, yet work on sexual dysfunctions and disjunctions due to unconscious conflict has not been sufficiently integrated into marital therapy but has been split off to be dealt with in behavioural approaches'. Scharff and Scharff (1991: 4) also say that the treatment of the sexual dysfunction 'cannot get far without considering the marital relationship because sexual problems express and give access to difficulties in relating that stem from unconscious factors'.

The time has therefore come for a re-evaluation of the relevance of psychodynamic thinking to sexual problems; this follows on from a considerable length of time when other perspectives have been dominant. This book carries out such a re-evaluation and puts forward developments in understanding that will help psychodynamic practitioners become more effective in applying their particular approach to sexual difficulties. Examples are given throughout, using cases from our own practice. In order to safeguard confidentiality in these case examples identities have been disguised, and material from more than one case has been merged. This process has been carried out in a way that safeguards the integrity of the examples, the explanations and the underlying psychodynamics.

Inevitably the main focus is on the ways sexual problems are viewed and treated in contemporary Western society; we include gay and lesbian issues, other sexual preferences and issues of sexual diversity. However, some attention is also given to the beliefs and needs of different ethnic groups. This book is inevitably written within a political context, in particular the continuing process of professionalization of counselling and psychotherapy. This includes not only the particular influences of the British Association of Counselling, the United Kingdom Council for Psychotherapy and the British Confederation of Psychotherapists, but also the larger context of the purchaser/ provider context for services. Additionally there are the important effects of continuing changes of policy on health services made by central government, as well as the developments in drug treatments for sexual difficulties.

In this book the terms *counselling, psychotherapy* and *therapy* are used interchangeably. The same applies to *counsellor, psychotherapist* and *therapist*. The word *client* is used throughout except where the relationship with a medical practitioner is referred to, where *patient* is preferred.

Chapter 1

The nature of sexual problems

Working with sexual problems requires specific knowledge of sexuality and sexual functioning. Scharff and Scharff (1991: 4) point out that, over the years, psychoanalytic therapies have struggled to address such problems without the benefit of the necessary knowledge about sexual functioning and dysfunctions. Sexual problems often bridge the artificial division that has been made between physical and psychological problems. This is a result of the way that sexual functioning and the personality as a whole interrelate, and the fact that sexual functioning is impinged upon by both internal and external factors. In the face of this complexity it is not surprising that the therapeutic approaches that have been developed to deal with sexual difficulties vary greatly in their focus.

This chapter outlines the anatomy and physiology of sexual response in men and women, looking particularly at the differences and similarities. While the sections on anatomy and physiology are primarily concerned with describing the external and internal genitalia, it is important to note that the whole body is involved in sexual behaviour and response. Stimulating many parts of the body can bring erotic pleasure to the giver and receiver, men and women, whatever their sexual orientation. The sections that follow suggest how the interaction of biological, intrapsychic, interpersonal relationships and cultural issues contributes in varying ways to sexual difficulties, and discuss how our conceptualizing and understanding of sexual problems is influenced by these factors.

Women's attitudes to their physical sexuality

Women are sometimes not very familiar or comfortable with their physical sexuality. Cultural ignorance and myths about sex and women's sexuality are part of the double standards that have throughout history granted greater sexual freedom to men than women. In our society sexuality has been particularly problematic for women, and Vance has identified how the socialization of women influences their ability to be sexual beings:

> Women – socialized by mothers to keep their dresses down, their pants up, and their bodies away from strangers – come to experience their own sexual impulses as dangerous. Self control and watchfulness become major and necessary female virtues. As a result, female desire is suspect from its first tingle . . . questionable until proven safe, and frequently too expensive when evaluated within the larger cultural framework . . . which poses the question: is it really worth it?
>
> (Vance 1984: 232–3)

However, during the last thirty years, perspectives on women's sexuality and sexual needs have undergone considerable change, as part of a more general process of a transformation in attitudes towards women. As a result, women have been able to begin to think differently about their sexuality. The advent of the freely available contraceptive pill, together with the notion that reproduction to some extent can be controlled, has freed sexual needs from such an intrinsic connection to childbearing.

In addition, during the 1970s the women's movement began to challenge and re-evaluate long-held beliefs about what sex means for women. This included demystifying women's bodies by encouraging women to talk together, to share experiences, and to gain wider access to information. This process has revealed that feelings about sex are often part of a complex and uneasy relationship that women can have with their bodies. In turn this generates in women fear and ignorance about the bodily changes and developments that occur throughout their life cycle. This has made it difficult for some women to express their sexuality and sexual needs in a non-stereotypical way.

Over time in Western societies information about sex and sexual practices has become more freely available and has helped to create a climate where discussion about sex and sexuality is more permissible. Women have in this context been able to challenge formulaic notions about their sexuality and to become more aware of their sexual needs. However, it has not all been gain, as the focus of the mass media on sexual issues has tended to create another set of stereotypes, which have created new pressures on women. One of these is an image of a heterosexual woman who has a perfect body, achieves orgasm easily, is successful in both her family and her career, and is able to juggle deftly the demands of home and work. Another more negative image is of the unfeminine woman who is gay because she is not attractive enough to lure a man. Her sexual attachment to other women is thereby portrayed as a second-best choice. Such stereotypes promote particular kinds of sexuality and pressurize women generally into aiming for unrealistic sexual goals. Such undermining of the ability of women to define their own sexuality leaves women feeling inadequate, whatever their sexual orientation, and also fails to recognize the kind of support that women need to define themselves (Kitzinger 1983: 76–7).

Women's sexual geography

Starting externally, the first most noticeable feature on an adult women is her pubic hair, which grows from the fatty tissue called

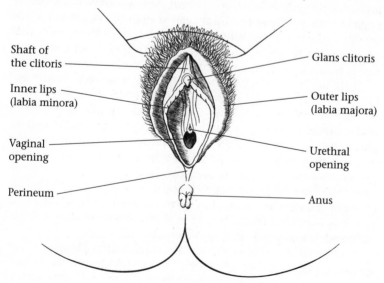

Figure 1.1 The external genitalia of the female

the *mons*. The mons area lies over the *pubic symphysis*, the joint of the pubic bone; some women feel this protruding slightly during sex. The outer genitals are called the *vulva*: there are two sets of vaginal lips, the inner (*labia minora*), and the outer (*labia majora*), which normally fold together over the entrance, but open during sexual arousal when they swell and change colour. The size and shape of the outer lips varies enormously between women. The area from the inner lips to the anus is called the *perineum*.

Outside the vagina and above it the inner lips join to form a soft fold of skin or hood, and there the *glans clitoris* is situated. This has a rich supply of sensory nerve endings, which makes it the most sensitive spot in the genital area. Some women find indirect contact of the clitoris more pleasurable than direct contact, which can be painful, especially when the woman is not aroused. The clitoris is one of a number of structures that are involved in the experience of orgasm. During sexual arousal the whole pelvic area, which has an extensive system of connecting veins, becomes firm and filled with blood. This process of vaso-congestion leads to changes in the colour of the vagina and causes it to swell. It produces a feeling of fullness and heaviness in the pelvic area, which women sometimes also experience just before menstruation when a similar physiological process is taking place. Just below, where the inner lips are attached to the underside of the clitoris, the opening for the bladder is situated. During sex women can feel pressure on the bladder, especially if

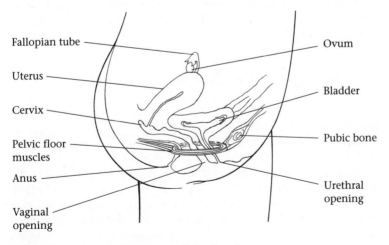

Figure 1.2 The sexual anatomy of the female

it is full. The *vagina* itself is capable of expansion and is composed of walls of soft muscle tissue that separate when anything is inserted. The walls of the vagina can vary from being almost dry to very wet; this will vary in sensitivity from woman to woman. It tends to be less moist before puberty, after menopause, or for some women just after their 'monthly' menstruation finishes. The vagina is likely to be more moist around ovulation and during pregnancy. In particular it becomes wet as a result of sexual arousal, when the vagina also swells. These secretions provide lubrication for sexual activity, and are sometimes the first sign of sexual excitement.

At the top of the vagina is the *cervix*, which is the neck of the uterus or the womb. In the cervix is a small passage through which sperm can pass. The uterus changes position and shape during the menstrual cycle, and during sexual excitement, and as a result the position of the cervix can alter slightly. The non-pregnant uterus is the size of a fist; extending outwards and back from the upper end are the two *fallopian tubes*. At either end lie the *ovaries*, which, apart from producing eggs, play an important part in the production of female sex hormones. Three groups of pelvic muscles are important in providing support for the organs in the pelvic area. Some of the muscles are situated about half-way up the woman's vagina, others around the entrance to the vagina. These muscles can contract involuntarily in a way which prevents intercourse or the insertion of tampons, or a speculum: this is a condition called *vaginismus*, which we discuss in detail later. The intentional contraction of these muscles during sexual stimulation can enhance a woman's sexual response, and in some cultures women are taught to do this for this purpose (see Strong *et al.* 1996: 68–9).

Men's attitudes to their physical sexuality

Despite the fact that men's sexual responses (as with women) involve the whole body and not just the genitals, the focus of sexuality and sexual practice is often on a man's penis, its size, and its relationship to ideas about masculinity. For example, many people believe that the size of a man's penis is directly related to his aggressiveness, sexual ability or sexual attractive-ness. Others believe that there is a relationship between the size of a man's penis and the size of his hand, foot, thumb, or nose (Strong *et al.* 1996: 92, 100). Furthermore there is a common belief that men are always ready for genital sex, and will never turn down an opportunity. In contrast, the facts are that size of the penis is not specifically related to body size, weight, muscular structure, race, ethnicity or sexual orientation; it is, rather, determined by individual heredity factors.

Masters and Johnson (1966) in their research discovered that there was no relationship between penis size and a man's ability to have sexual intercourse or to satisfy his partner. The sexual anatomy of all men is structurally the same, but there is considerable variation in the appearance of their genitals and in their need for sex. The culturally sanctioned myths and misconceptions about men's sexual anatomy and sexual needs have encouraged both men and women to develop a preoccupation with fantasies about genitals and sexual capacity. The consequences of this for men can be the creation of unrealistic expectations and a consequent reduction of self-esteem.

Men's sexual geography

The *penis* is composed of a base and a main body, and varies in length from man to man. It nearly always looks shorter than it actually is to the man himself, as he generally views his penis from above. From this perspective the man sees his pubic hair, and the shaft of the penis foreshortened, with his testes lying either side. The head of the penis in the uncircumcised man is covered by the foreskin, which is retractable. The shaft of the penis contains three cylinders of erectile tissue: a pair of *corpora cavernosa* (cavernous bodies) lying parallel to each other, and (below) the *corpus spongiosum* (spongy body). These cylinders contain smooth muscle tissue and vascular spaces that inflate with blood during an erection.

The structure of these tissues are of central importance in the mechanism of erection. Engorgement of the corpus spongiosum occurs during an erection and happens in such a way that the urethra which it contains is still able to pass semen. The tip of the corpus spongiosum expands to form a bulb, and is the site for the opening of the urethra. This bulb is known as the *glans penis* and is particularly important in sexual arousal because it is richly supplied with sensory nerve endings. This makes it especially responsive to stimulation, although some men find a direct touch painful when they are aroused. The base of the glans expands to form a ridge with the shaft of the penis. This ridge is

(a) uncircumcised penis   (b) circumcised penis

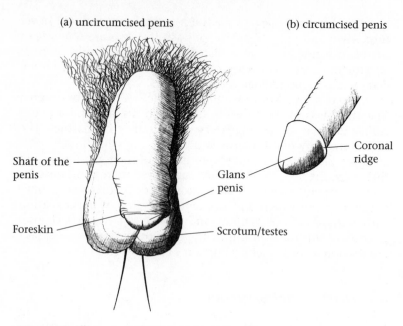

Shaft of the
penis

Foreskin

Coronal
ridge

Glans
penis

Scrotum/testes

Figure 1.3   The external genitalia of the male

called the *coronal ridge*. In the uncircumcised penis the glans is
covered by a double layer of skin – the *prepuce*, or foreskin.

At the base of the penis lies a pouch of skin called the
scrotum, which is sensitive to the touch, and contains the *testes*,
which lie either side of the base of the penis. These can be slightly
different in size, and one generally hangs a little lower than the
other. The skin of the scrotum can vary in appearance because
during sexual arousal, or when the man is cold or anxious, the
testicles are pulled close to the body, causing the skin to wrinkle
and become more compact. These changes help maintain a constant temperature within the testes so sperm can be produced.
Within each testicle are millions of tiny seminiferous tubules that
produce sperm. The testes also produce the male sex hormone,
testosterone. On the outer side of each testicle is attached the *epididymis*, which consists of a collection of coiled tubes to receive
sperm. The *vas deferens* is a long fibromuscular tube leading from
each epididymis to the *prostate*, along which sperm pass to be
stored in the *ampulla*. It is the vas deferens that is cut in carrying out a vasectomy.

The prostate gland is about the size of a chestnut, and lies
below the bladder with the urethra passing through it. Some
of the fluid contained in semen is provided by the prostate,

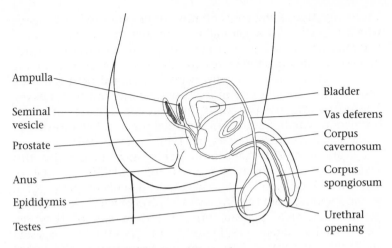

Figure 1.4 The sexual anatomy of the male

although most of the secretions are produced by the *seminal vesicles*, two elongated sacs which lie behind the bladder and the prostate gland. The fluid is discharged down along the ejaculatory duct into the prostatic part of the urethra, where it joins the sperm that have been stored in the *ampulla*. A few drops of fluid may appear at the tip of the penis before ejaculation and at the early stages of arousal. For some men this can be a source of embarrassment if the drops are excessive, though the amount varies between individuals. This fluid is usually clear, unlike semen which is cloudy, and it is thought that it comes from a gland just below the prostate, the function of which is unknown. It can, however, contain sperm, a fact that couples need to be aware of in avoiding conception.

Sexual arousal and sexual response

Even though the sexual anatomies of men and women are distinctly different, the pattern of sexual response is similar. One clear difference is that men often, though not always, become more quickly physically aroused than women. Another is that some women can have one or more further orgasms after the first, in contrast to men, who have to wait a period of time before it becomes physically possible. For both females and males, the physiological changes that occur during sexual arousal are dependent on two processes: vasocongestion and myotonia.

Vasocongestion is the concentration of blood in the body tissue which happens in the genital area, causing the genitals to swell and change colour, the erect penis being an obvious sign of this process. Myotonia is the increased muscle tension accompanying the increase in blood flow. If orgasm is attained then the body goes through involuntary muscle contractions and then relaxes. The sexual response pattern is the same for all forms of sexual behaviour, whether autoerotic or coital, or in a heterosexual or homosexual context (Masters and Johnson 1966, 1970).

Various models have been put forward to describe this sexual response pattern, the most influential being that of Masters and Johnson (1966). This model described four stages of sexual response from the physical and physiological changes that occur; excitement, plateau, orgasm and resolution. However, others such as Kaplan (1977) and Stuntz (1988) have suggested an additional stage – desire – at the beginning of the sexual response pattern, and this has generally been followed by later writers. Desire can be triggered both by external cues (such as sight, smell, taste or sound) and internal cues (for instance thoughts, fantasies, and the need or drive created for sex by emotional states such as happiness). As such these thoughts and feelings activate excitement and the corresponding sexual arousal responses that prepare the body for sexual activity. Understanding how the sexual response pattern operates has had a great effect on how sexual problems are classified, as we shall see in the next chapter. We take the view that sexual desire is a necessary prerequisite for sexual arousal to occur, but others claim that sexual desire can be a response to being sexually aroused.

Sexual desire problems frequently present clinically, and may be described by clients in various ways. Some claim that either their own or their partner's sexual interest is too high or too low, judged in relation to some idea of what is normal. Other couples, who are more aware of the wide possible range of sexual interest, may conceptualize their problem more as a discrepancy between their levels of desire. The pattern of sexual response of men and women is summarized below using the four-stage model of Masters and Johnson as a guide, with the addition at the beginning of the sexual desire phase.

Sexual desire

Sexual desire is a fundamental aspect of sexual functioning because it produces the motivation and inclination towards feeling and acting sexual. It exists biologically, where it is under the influence of constitutional differences including hormonal, anatomical and neurophysiological factors, and also as an emotional and psychological energy that is relationship seeking. Consequent on the latter, sexual desire is profoundly shaped by the individual's intrapsychic issues and their relationships with others, including the society in which they live. These factors contribute to the complexity of sexual experience, and means that aspects of sexual desire may play a part in what might seem to be a disruption rooted later in the response cycle.

Excitement phase

During this stage sexual arousal develops further in response to continued sexual stimulation. It marks the start of the physical and physiological changes, and may last from several minutes to several hours. The general process of arousal is accompanied by bodily reactions in both sexes, namely increases in heart rate and blood pressure, skin changes and muscle tension. For women, within half a minute of effective stimulation the vagina becomes moist with the lubricant produced from tissue in the vaginal walls. As the extra blood pulses through these tissues the walls of the vagina swell and open up instead of resting on each other, making the shape of a tent. The outer vaginal lips draw apart as a result of the increased blood flow, and the inner lips swell with the extra blood. The increased flow of blood affects the uterus, which expands and starts to lift up and tilts forward from the pelvic floor muscles. In some women the clitoris becomes erect, as it swells and the hood retracts.

In men the excitement phase involves the combination of penile arterial dilation, increased arterial blood, and the constriction of the blood outflow. This is followed by the active relaxation of the smooth muscle tissue of the corpora cavernosa. These processes enable the penis to become engorged and erect. The foreskin retracts, the scrotal sac tightens and the testes are elevated. Secretions from the Cowper glands sometimes appear at the tip of the penis.

Plateau phase

According to Masters and Johnson this is a period in which the responses of the excitement phase continue up to a point of ejaculatory inevitability for men and to the brink of orgasm for women. Some authors believe this is a continuation of the excitement phase; as such it is not a distinct phase in itself and does not warrant a separate reference (Jehu 1979).

Orgasm phase

The sexual response cycle reaches a peak for men and women with an intensely pleasurable experience called an orgasm. Women who experience orgasms describe sensations that often come in waves of feeling as their pelvic floor muscles, vagina and uterus contract rhythmically. This is often preceded by a sense of orgasmic inevitability, where the woman's physiological changes coalesce and lead to the experience of orgasm as part of that chain of events. It is believed that this occurs because the extreme vasocongestion of the genital area, in particular the clitoris, triggers a neural reflex which creates the sensations that make the muscles in the vagina and pelvic area involuntarily contract. Because the female sexual response cycle does not include a refractory period, it is possible for women to experience further orgasms.

For men the orgasm phase is marked by the two separate stages of emission and expulsion. These are preceded by a distinct sense of ejaculatory inevitability, a point at which ejaculation will occur without any further stimulation and therefore cannot be prevented. Men with premature ejaculation are often unaware when they are approaching this point because of their rapid sexual responses. The sense of ejaculatory inevitability is believed to result from the contraction of the prostate gland and the seminal vesicles, which in turn causes the contents to be discharged into the prostatic urethra. Emission is brought about by contractions in the epididymis, vas deferens, seminal vesicle and prostate, during which the internal sphincter of the bladder is closed. This closure prevents retrograde ejaculation and leakage of urine into the urethra during ejaculation.

The subjective experiences of orgasm begin at the emission stage and the sensation of orgasm is at its most intense during ejaculation. There is evidence that the intensity of sensation may be related to the volume of ejaculate, which has been linked to the interval between ejaculations, larger volumes being recorded after periods of abstinence. The subjective pleasure and intensity of each orgasm is also related to the degree of receptivity or state of mind prior to orgasm, as well as to the intensity and duration of sexual arousal.

Resolution phase

The final phase is that of resolution, when the anatomical and physiological changes associated with the earlier part of the cycle are reversed, and the body returns to an unaroused state. This resolution takes place more slowly if there has been no orgasm. For men the resolution phase takes place in a more gradual way than for women, as the penis loses tumescence, and this may be further delayed if there has been prolonged stimulation during the excitement phase. Following this there is a refractory period during which erection and orgasm is not possible. Over a man's life cycle this period of time may vary from a few minutes in adolescence to days in the elderly, and partly depends on the physical health of the individual.

The orgasm debate

The female orgasm has been the subject of debate and controversy since the early part of the twentieth century, when Freud put forward a distinction between the role of the clitoris and the vagina in the psychosexual development of women. Freud hypothesized that women had two main erotogenic zones, the clitoris and the vagina. Erotic activity in the earliest stages of development centres around the clitoris, and ideally there is a subsequent transition of erotic response to the vagina. From this people have inferred that Freud makes this distinction with the implication that the vaginal orgasm produced by intercourse is more 'mature', and is evidence of normal psychosexual development. In contrast, clitoral orgasm is seen as evidence that a woman is fixated at an earlier stage of development. The work of researchers carrying out laboratory studies, in particular that of Masters and Johnson, revealed no distinction between different types of orgasm. In fact, not only was the incorrectness of such theories demonstrated, but evidence gathered to the contrary. The clitoris may always be crucial in the female orgasmic response, however women experience their orgasms. This whole debate has served to distract attention from other important areas of discussion about the female experience of sex, and has unduly restricted the focus of sexual response to what happens in the genital area.

   The cultural emphasis on orgasm as the primary indicator of sexual satisfaction for women excludes those who, for whatever reason, never have an orgasm, and those who do not feel the need for them on every occasion. Currently it is believed that about 10 per cent of women cannot have an orgasm from any sexual activity, even if they are highly aroused. However, whether a woman is orgasmic, multi-orgasmic or non-orgasmic is no indication of sexual satisfaction, which is an entirely subjective experience. This point is made by Kitzinger in her discussion of the debate about female orgasm when she says that genital sex 'is just one small part of this rich experience. Reducing sex to something limited to what happens to a clitoris is to drain from it much of what makes female sexuality exciting and alive . . . It is time we re-assessed the widespread assumptions as to the overriding importance of genital sex in our lives' (Kitzinger 1983: 26).

Hormonal aspects of sexual response

For both men and women the physiology of the sexual response cycle involves a complex interaction of thoughts and feelings, sensory perceptions (central and peripheral), neural responses – and the presence of hormones. The sex drive in both men and women is biologically influenced by the hormone testosterone. Women produce much less of this than men but are more sensitive to its effects. The relationship between testosterone level and sexual interest is not fully understood. Changes in testosterone levels do not always produce a subsequent change in levels of sexual interest or functioning. In women oestrogens help maintain a healthy vagina and lubrication, benefits that can be reduced during the menopause. As the role of hormones in sexual function is not fully understood it is important that sexual problems that may have a hormonal basis are properly investigated and assessed.

Medical and psychiatric aspects of sexual problems

Sexual problems have a complex and interactive relationship with medical and psychiatric conditions and their treatment. Apart from the effects on the genitals, which we have described in detail, various other parts of the body are involved in sexual response, including the cerebral cortex and the limbic system of the brain, the nervous system and the endocrine glands. Any disruption in these areas of the body resulting from illness and accidents, or problem mental states consequent on personal or relationships difficulties, can have a direct effect on a person's ability to function sexually.

It is important in all forms of psychological assessment and treatment that full consideration is given to the possibility of underlying causes that need medical attention. Illness can be conceptualized as an unexpected and unwelcome process of change to which adjustment needs to be made (see Jones *et al.* 1995). Many people use a process of denial and work on the assumption that illness, accidents and disability are things that happen to other people. Such processes of denial are not wholly negative and enable us to control anxiety about the unpredictability of life. Chronic or serious illness therefore usually brings a need for extensive psychological as well as practical adjustment. Part of this adjustment is to the kinds of sexual and relationship problems that can arise.

Almost any illness can have an effect on sexual functioning. For example, having a bad cold or flu is likely to decrease sexual interest to a degree in most people. With most minor illnesses in most people these effects are minor and transient. Nevertheless, there are illnesses, disabilities and treatments that have a more damaging effect on normal sexual functioning, either directly or indirectly. The most direct way is through disrupting, or making physically painful or uncomfortable, physical sexual functioning. The main indirect disturbances come through decreasing libido, disturbing body image and altering roles within couple relationships. It is important to look at effects in two categories: those that are likely to be associated with any chronic illness, and those that arise from particular conditions.

Sometimes sexual activity is impinged upon by medical conditions or treatments affecting the sexual areas of the body. Examples of this are thrush and urinary infections, and some sexually transmitted diseases that can affect the genitals, and cysts and tumours in the anus. Any conditions affecting the blood or nerve supply to the genitals are likely to disrupt sexual functioning, especially in men. Therefore spinal injuries can cause disturbance of erection, lack of sensation and lack of orgasm. Various neurological disorders, such as multiple sclerosis, can produce erectile and ejaculatory problems.

Diabetes can result in erectile problems in men and a lowering of sexual responsiveness in women, probably as a result of nerve damage. The ability to have an erection is very dependent on an efficient blood supply, and so arterial disease and hypertension can result in erectile dysfunction. There are a number of disorders that make sexual activity painful or uncomfortable, of which arthritis is one of the most common. Drugs can disrupt sexual functioning through various mechanisms, and the most common groups of drugs that do this include anti-hypertensive and psychiatric drugs. Surgery in the pelvic area can result in nerve damage that affects functioning and sensation. Therefore counsellors must take into account the side effects of past and current medical treatments in both the psychological and physical arenas.

We have already noted that any illness can produce a loss of libido simply through the loss of feelings of well-being. The most common states of mind associated with chronic or serious illness are depression and anxiety. Both of these normally decrease sexual interest and of course can exist for reasons other than physical illness. Chronic illnesses also reduce libido through tiredness, while the presence of uncontrolled pain is also important. Certain drugs, such as anti-depressants and tranquillizers, often decrease sexual interest.

A good body image is an important prerequisite for satisfactory sex. It is hard to feel positively about sharing one's body with another person if one is unhappy about it. Illness and surgery can disrupt body image through their impact on external appearance and in more subtle ways. Examples that affect external appearance are mastectomy, colostomy or ileostomy, and scarring. Less direct causes of a deterioration in body image are hysterectomy, cancer and the knowledge that one has a major illness. Generally in illness, feelings of self-worth and attractiveness to others are threatened at a time when there can be a great need for intimacy. In this situation the loss of satisfying sexual relating is also the loss of a means of comfort and the reduction of tension at a time when both of these are very much needed.

For some couples difficulties in their sexual relationship seem trivial in the light of an illness. For others their sexual relationship takes on a new importance and they are keen to obtain help with sexual problems. Health challenges can threaten the stability of close relationships, and there is evidence that the rate of break up of relationships may double in the face of seriously chronic health problems. However, there is also evidence that through periods of illness some relationships can be preserved, effectively restructured or even improved (Jones *et al.* 1995). We return to the topic of medical and psychiatric issues in Chapter 5, in the context of assessment.

The psychosomatic circle of sex

Bancroft describes sexual function as a process which is 'par excellence psychosomatic' (1989: 12) and offers a model that links different aspects of the experience. He says that in order to have a satisfactory sexual experience there are certain basic requirements, which include the need to feel comfortable about the body and the physiological changes that occur during sexual arousal. Sexual activity also presupposes the ability to become vulnerable by lowering psychological defences. The whole body is involved in the interplay of physical and psychological processes, with each component part relying on communication and feedback from the other. Successful interaction of these elements enables the person to have a satisfactory sexual experience, but also means that failure in any one part of the circle can lead to sexual difficulties.

The psychosomatic circle of sex identifies the interplay between the psychological and somatic elements that are involved in the sexual arousal cycle of events. It is important to note that sexual arousal can be enhanced or lowered depending on the feedback and communication between the different parts of the system. These are identified in Figure 1.5. This shows how the mental processes involved in the conscious and unconscious mind interpret bodily arousal and allow for links to be made between the physical and emotional state of arousal. These links help to create the necessary physiological basis for sexual arousal to occur. Moving on to the brain, mechanisms such as the limbic system help to mediate this arousal through the central nervous system and through the spinal cord and local reflexes. In turn these nerve pathways help control the ability of the genitals to inflate with blood and experience sensation. The unconscious mind has been added to Bancroft's original schema because it is often unprocessed experiences, memories or defensive processes that are activated which can interfere with arousal. Successful sexual arousal ultimately depends on the interaction between the individual's biological and psychological systems.

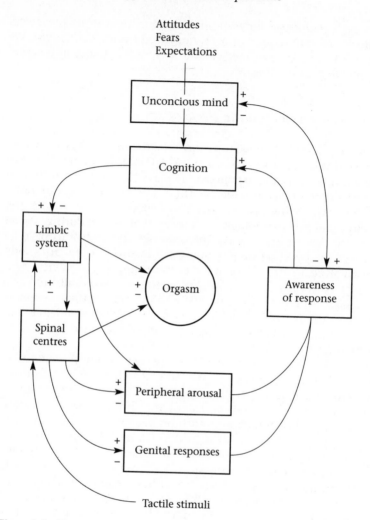

Figure 1.5 The psychosomatic circle of sex (after Bancroft 1989)

Conclusion

Sexuality is a complex area of experience, and these complexities often surface abruptly when individuals have to make sense of the nature and meaning of sexual difficulties. Those helping clients with sexual problems need to be able to understand the influence of a range of interrelated factors on the individual's ability to be sexual. Disturbances in sexual functioning may have either organic or psychological origins (or both), but inevitably the effects are experienced at a number of different levels: biologically, interpsychically and intrapersonally.

For our purposes it is important to reassert that physiological processes can be interfered with and inhibited by conscious and unconscious psychological processes. The biological characteristics that are involved in sexual arousal are accompanied by cognitions that give meaning and understanding to this experience. Internal psychological processes are influenced by the spectrum of social, intrapsychic and relationship factors which can precipitate conscious and unconscious reactions to the sexual experience. Psychodynamic theories consider these internal processes to be central to the way people function. In Chapter 3 we look at these aspects in more detail, but before that, in the next chapter, we consider the principal presenting sexual problems.

Chapter 2

The main sexual problems

Issues in the classification of sexual problems

The treatment of sexual problems is directly affected by the way that they are classified. Within psychoanalysis sexual problems have been seen as a manifestation of an underlying psychopathology, and their treatment as the resolution of the underlying conflicts within the personality. However, the last twenty years of research into sexual difficulties has demonstrated the need for a variety of approaches, in response to the multiple factors involved in their genesis and persistence. Masters and Johnson developed a classification system that reflected their understanding of the sexual response cycle, a system followed by others such as Kaplan. The most commonly used classification of sexual problems organizes them under the headings of 'women's problems' and 'men's problems'. Within this division problems are identified at certain points in the sexual response cycle, and thereby linked with the aspect of sexual function affected by the problem. Therefore the main female problems are described as impaired sexual interest, lack of arousal, orgasmic dysfunction, vulval pain, vaginismus, dyspareunia and sexual phobias. Correspondingly, the main male problems are erectile dysfunction, premature ejaculation, retarded and non-ejaculation, impaired sexual interest and, less commonly, sexual phobias and psychogenic pain.

One of the objections to this classification is that it does not recognize sufficiently the commonality in sexual response between men and women. In the 1970s Kaplan added to the classification schema by distinguishing between sexual desire, sexual arousal (excitement) and orgasm. In this schema the main headings become disorders of sexual interest, disorders of arousal and disorders of orgasm. She identifies hypoactive sexual desire as a common problem for both sexes, although it tends to present in women as a problem for treatment more commonly than in men. For women, disorders of arousal include not feeling physically aroused, and lubrication problems; while for men, erectile dysfunction is the main difficulty of this kind. Orgasmic dysfunction in women is typically a difficulty or inability to experience orgasm. In men it describes a group of disorders such as premature ejaculation, retarded ejaculation and ejaculatory pain. One drawback of this classification is that there are a number of conditions that do not fit into it, and are collected together as 'other types of dysfunction': dyspareunia in women, pain on intercourse in men, vaginismus in women, and sexual phobias in men and women.

Both forms of classification suffer from the limitations of the perspectives that have informed them, which are predominantly medical and behavioural. This has led to important aspects of sexual problems being sidelined, in particular the interactive elements. Consequently the problem tends to be located solely in one partner. What might be described from one point of view as one partner's lack of interest in sex may be also conceptualized as a problem of *difference in interest in sex*. Similarly, in other instances, the underlying issue may be a difficulty in communicating about sex or a general relationship problem. The process of classification inevitably emphasizes one dimension of the problem. For example, a categorization by life stage highlights teenage years as being characterized by premature ejaculation in men and vaginismus in women. The predominant occurrence of erectile dysfunction appears in middle and old age.

We have seen how various assumptions and philosophies underlie the various ways of describing and classifying sexual problems. In general the fact that sexual problems can have a physical cause has led, in their description and classification, to an overemphasis on their physical characteristics. As a result the general population are led to see their sexual functioning in an over-physical way. It is possible to include a greater psychological dimension in categorization, using such ideas as sexual dissatisfaction, sexual frustration and incompatibility in interest. The possibilities of developing a schema focusing on the underlying psychodynamic processes involved are of particular relevance to our current purposes. We shall return to this in Chapter 4.

The conventional classification of sexual problems

Accepting these reservations, the conventional *problems in women/problems in men* classification serves as an introduction to information about the main sexual problems that present for treatment. In conceptualizing and treating these from a psychodynamic perspective we seek to move away from the limi-tations and disadvantages of this arrangement, including an additional category of sexual problems manifesting primarily in a relationship.

It is important to be aware of a common distinction in describing sexual problems as *primary* and *secondary*. Primary problems are those that have always existed in sexual relation-ships, and secondary ones are those that began at a particular point following satisfactory functioning. Another useful distinc-tion that can also usefully be made is between total or pervasive problems that occur in all contexts, and situational ones that occur only in a particular context or contexts. In considering the list in Table 2.1, it is important to distinguish sexual dysfunction and sexual dissatisfaction. The degree of sexual satisfaction that an individual experiences is affected by a number of factors, not least satisfaction with the rest of the relationship. Sexual dys-function is tolerated by many couples if the rest of their rela-tionship is good.

Table 2.1 shows how sexual dysfunction is described in the standard manual used by psychiatrists; Table 2.2 gives the con-ventional classification used by sex therapists, also used in the discussion of sexual problems that follows.

Sexual problems in women

Impaired sexual interest

Loss of sexual interest is the most frequent presenting sexual problem by couples in sex therapy clinics (Schover and LoPiccolo 1982). As Hawton (1985) reports, this usually presents as a female

Table 2.1 Sexual dysfunction as described in *The Classification of Mental and Behavioural Disorders (ICD-10)* (World Health Organization 1992: 32)

Relevant category: 'Sexual dysfunction not caused by organic disease or disorder'

Definition: 'Sexual dysfunction covers the various ways in which an individual is unable to participate in a sexual relationship as he or she would wish'

Classification of presentations:
• lack or loss of sexual desire (as a primary problem rather than a secondary result of another problem)
• sexual aversion and lack of sexual enjoyment
• premature ejaculation
• excessive sexual drive
• other sexual dysfunction not caused by organic disorder or disease
• failure of genital response (inc. erectile dysfunction and lack of vaginal lubrication)
• orgasmic dysfunction
• nonorganic vaginismus
• nonorganic dyspareunia
• unspecified sexual dysfunction not caused by organic disorder or disease

Table 2.2 Classification of sexual problems

Sexual problems in women
• impaired sexual interest
• lack of arousal
• orgasmic dysfunction
• vaginismus
• dyspareunia including vulval pain
• sexual phobias

Sexual problems in men
• erectile dysfunction
• premature ejaculation
• retarded and non-ejaculation
• impaired sexual interest
• sexual phobias
• pain

Sexual problems manifesting primarily in a relationship
• differences of interest in sex
• difficulties in communicating about sex
• a general relationship difficulty causing a sexual problem

problem, accounting for 52 per cent of women but only 6 per cent of men in his sample of couples. This is the most common problem in women seeking help and includes a wide range of difficulties. For example, some women lack any spontaneous interest, but can get aroused and enjoy sexual activity once they become involved. This may reflect differences in how men and women have been socialized to take different roles when initiating sex, as in the past men in heterosexual relationships were encouraged to see themselves as the initiator of sex, in contrast to the women's role, which was to respond and to be available. In this way differences in sexual interest may well have been masked in the past. An alternative form of impaired sexual interest is where the woman has an initial spontaneous interest which is lost once sexual activity begins. This can be perhaps best conceptualized as a difficulty in carrying through an interest in the possibility of sexual activity to the physicality of sexual activity.

In assessing impaired sexual interest it is important to take into account the wide range of interest characteristic of women generally, the woman's previous level of interest, and whether the woman herself thinks she has a problem. In many instances important background influences are negative attitudes to sex from significant others in early life, often resulting in negative body image. Often sexual interest changes following particular life events. Examples of these are childbirth and the hormonal changes associated with a woman's menstrual cycle. Changes in sexual interest are understandably often related to concurrent difficulties such as depression or a poor relationship with the woman's partner. It rarely has a direct physical cause, but can be a consequence of any chronic illness or disability. All these factors affect a woman's libido, and must be taken into account in assessing such presentations.

Lack of arousal

One of the specific physical signs of low arousal is lack of lubrication and vaginal swelling. The physiological responses are halted by a lack of sexual excitement, which may in turn be affected by a whole host of factors outlined above. The cause for this is usually psychological, such as when a block on sexual arousal is a defence against feeling sexual, in order to avoid guilt or other negative feelings. Important considerations centre around the woman's attitude to sex and her previous sexual experiences.

Orgasmic dysfunction

The enjoyment of sexual activity without reaching an orgasm is not necessarily a problem. Probably between one third and one half of sexually active women never experience an orgasm on intercourse without additional stimulation, and many women only have an orgasm occasionally. It is important to ascertain whether or not the woman is able to have orgasms in other situations, i.e. with masturbation, or with different techniques. Unrealistic expectations and goals can be adopted from the media or be the result of pressure from a partner. Orgasm has been set up by our culture as something women must strive for and which their sexual partners are entitled to expect. Discovering one's own sexual needs and ability to respond is difficult in the face of internal and external pressure to achieve certain goals. Clearly difficulties with orgasm may be associated with either impaired interest or lack of arousal, and the underlying factors that affect them.

Vaginismus

This describes the situation where intercourse is painful or impossible because of spasm in the muscles surrounding the entrance to the vagina when penetration is attempted. It is an automatic response over which the woman feels she has no control. The problem can be a mild or transient one when women begin sexual intercourse and are anxious about it. Alternatively it can be a longer-term problem more associated with a fear of penetration. In this latter situation it is often a problem that has always existed for the woman. Commonly couples come for help with vaginismus when they want to conceive, and have been unable to consummate the relationship.

Secondary vaginismus often follows on from some traumatic physical or emotional experience. Examples are vaginal trauma (such as an episiotomy) and recurrent vaginal infections, as well as serious assaults such as rape and sexual abuse. Some women have a phobia about penetration, reflected in difficulties with tampons, extreme fears about childbirth and a distorted view of vagina size. Their vaginismus forms part of this phobic pattern and leads to the avoidance of penetration of any kind. However, many women with vaginismus enjoy other forms of sexual activity and are sexually responsive, often to the point of orgasm with manual or oral stimulation. In considering the possibility of vaginismus in a client, it is important to bear in mind that a dislike of penetrative sex is not necessarily an indication of a sexual problem but may be an expression of her sexual preferences.

Dyspareunia including vulval pain

Dyspareunia describes pain on intercourse and is often associated with poor sexual arousal and mild vaginismus. The causes of dyspareunia can be a complex mixture of psychological and organic factors. For example a localized vaginal infection can leave tenderness and inflammation at the entrance to the vagina and can make sexual intercourse painful. Even if the infection is treated, some women may still experience residual discomfort resulting from feelings of vulnerability and anxiety about that area of their body. These and more serious gynaecological conditions need to be addressed and excluded, especially if the woman reports persistent pain during intercourse. Examination and assessment by a doctor is always indicated if the woman has not previously consulted. In some women dyspareunia has occurred from their first sexual experience and persists due to their continued fear and inability to discuss with their partners their ambivalent feelings about sex. Sexual trauma and sexual abuse have also been indicated as the causes of dyspareunia and vulval pain problems (Roberts 1996).

Pain on intercourse can be the result of the lack of arousal and lubrication. Attempting penetrative sex without sufficient lubrication produces painful friction on sensitive tissues. Lubrication difficulties are also associated with hormonal changes at the menopause, when women's oestrogen levels drop, with resultant vaginal dryness. Pain on deep penetration can result from the penis thrusting against the cervix and the uterus, since with insufficient arousal the normal elevating of the reproductive internal organs cannot take place. Black (1988) compares this assault on the woman's organs to that of the man being kicked in the testes during coitus. The clinical evidence suggests that some women with deep dyspareunia lubricate and are sexually responsive to manual or oral stimulation, indicating that perhaps the difficulty occurs for women in the later stages of arousal. Emotional conflict, which may be unconscious, can lead to the inhibition of the processes that lead to vaginal expansion and uterine elevation (Hiller 1996).

Vulval pain is a term covering a group of difficulties which may or may not exist concurrently with the experience of dyspareunia. Recently there have been a number of advances in the understanding of pain syndromes that women experience in the vulval area. Some women describe dermatological problems that range from skin sensitivity to debilitating pain, conditions that are currently poorly understood and therefore have often not been treated appropriately. Untreated or chronic organic problems can lead to persistent physical, psychological and sexual difficulties for women, including depression and relationship difficulties. In some situations relationship problems may contribute to vulval pain, or produce it via sexual and psychodynamic processes.

Frequently vulval pain may be the persistent presenting problem in a relationship where the couple would otherwise be struggling in another way with issues related to intimacy. In these cases the problem needs to be approached from a couple as well as an individual perspective. Unfortunately many women have had inadequate help with these kinds of problems and have not had access to the kind of services that can look at the various biological, emotional, sexual and relational roots of these difficulties. Graziottin (1998) points out the need for competent medical and psychological assessment of women with these problems so that they are not left with a chronic untreated condition.

Sexual phobias

Sexual phobia or sexual aversion is a consistently phobic response to sexual activity or the idea of such activity. It can be confused with low desire, as avoidance often reveals itself as a lack of interest in sexual matters. However, sexual phobias are more of a defence against anxiety-causing situations, such as intimacy or touch. Sexual aversion may cause anxiety without any kind of sexual contact, whereby the thought of sex or any kind of associated physical contact leads to an extremely anxious reaction including sweating, diarrhoea and nausea. The persistence of such internalized reactions can lead to worries about being normal, or concerns about sexual orientation. As such, anticipating sex or an aspect of sexual activity can sometimes provoke a greater anxiety than physical sexual activity itself.

Sexual problems in men

Erectile dysfunction

This is the most common dysfunction among men seeking help. The range of disorders is considerable, the most common being loss of an erection on penetration. The erectile response is very vulnerable to disruption from both physical disorders and psychological influences, particularly anxiety. It is also a side effect of some drugs, including alcohol and long-term smoking. Erectile problems can be a consequence of chronic degenerative medical conditions such as diabetes or multiple sclerosis. These latter conditions affect the blood flow to the penis and cause vascular or peripheral nerve damage which can affect the ability of the penis to respond. Primary total erectile failure – where the man never gets erections, even during his sleep – is rare and usually has a physical basis. Where men present with secondary erectile dysfunction this is usually due to a combination of causative factors. A common situation is where a man finds it difficult to admit to having problems or worries about sex, which in turn generates a level of suppressed anxiety that inevitably affects physical functioning.

Cultural myths about male sexuality have led many men to believe that their sexual function is unfailingly dependable, and this includes the expectation that sexual need and response will remain the same throughout life. One result of this can be the development of performance anxiety, where the man gets caught up in a cycle of worries about his ability to perform sexually. This puts him under great pressure to produce an erection, which in turn inhibits his ability to have one. This can further lead to spectatoring, where the man becomes preoccupied with monitoring the degree of erection, which further interferes with the ability to become sexually aroused.

Performance anxiety is prevalent among gay men, where it may be a particular problem since many gay men 'move in a social, sexual milieu where sexual arousal is expected immediately or soon after meeting someone. If response is not rapidly forthcoming, rejection is likely' (Reece 1988: 46). Secondary situational erection difficulties are the most commonly presenting sub-group of this problem. This is the loss of erection on or during penetration for men who have had intercourse successfully in the past. Such problems often relate to unexpressed problems in the couple relationship, to internal conflicts, or to worries about sexual performance.

Premature ejaculation

This refers to a situation where lack of control of ejaculation leads to dissatisfaction for the man or his partner. Rapid ejaculation is common among men having their first sexual experiences and is usually a primary problem. Important factors are anxiety, early experiences of rapid masturbation, early intercourse in uncomfortable and or anxiety-producing situations, and stress. It can be a response to a partner's problem, such as pain on intercourse, and there is a causal relationship both ways with lack of interest and non-orgasm in women. Women who are not sexually responsive may encourage their partner to ejaculate quickly, and partners of men with premature ejaculation are not likely to become very aroused during intercourse. Men often try to deal with the problem by shortening foreplay or using distracting thoughts, both of which tend to make it worse!

There have been various ways in which premature ejaculation has been defined. Originally it was defined by the time between penetration and ejaculation, but such a definition is very arbitrary. Some have stated it exists where the man ejaculates before his partner has an orgasm, but this is very dependent on partner responsiveness as well as on other situational factors. A more useful definition focuses on the concepts of control and dissatisfaction, identifying whether the man feels he has control over when he ejaculates, and whether the point at which he ejaculates gives rise to lack of satisfaction for him or his partner.

Retarded and non-ejaculation

Delayed and absent ejaculation or orgasm is relatively uncommon. Again it is not easy to define as what 'delay' is acceptable, since this depends on a person's expectations. It is important to distinguish this problem from retrograde ejaculation, where the ejaculate goes into the bladder, a condition which is sometimes the result of prostate surgery or a side effect of particular medications such as certain anti-psychotic drugs. In this situation the man experiences orgasm but no ejaculation as the ejaculate is propelled backwards into the bladder, with the result that semen is passed in the urine. Inhibited or retarded ejaculation refers to a situation where, despite arousal and a firm erection, a man is unable to proceed to orgasm and ejaculation. This can occur in particular situations and circumstances, such as with a current partner during penetrative sex, whereas it may not happen during masturbation, or have occurred with a previous partner.

In some instances a man is able to have an orgasm without ejaculation, and some HIV-positive gay men have perfected this as a technique. This enables them to have anal sex without the intrusion of excessive worries about passing their virus to their partners. In heterosexual couples retarded and non-ejaculation commonly leads to concerns about conception, and sometimes this is the point at which couples ask for help. There are many psychological issues which can become associated with this problem, including the fear of the man's partner becoming pregnant, gender identity issues, hostility towards the partner and other relationship problems.

Impaired sexual interest

In discussing female problems we noted that in his sample of couples Hawton (1985) reports 52 per cent of women and 6 per cent of men as having loss of interest. The low incidence of requests for therapy by men could be for a number of reasons, not least that men's lack of interest often leads to performance difficulties, especially erectile failure. It may well be that many occurrences of impaired sexual interest in men are subsumed under this and other problems category headings later in the sexual response cycle, as a consequence of men's physiological response to sexual stimuli being more sensitive to lack of interest. Additionally the myths and stereotypes about men – that they are always interested in sex and ready for it – may make it difficult for men to acknowledge a loss of interest. Impaired sexual interest in men in heterosexual relationships can be difficult to assess because it can hide behind other presentations, such as erectile failure and low interest in their partners.

Sexual phobias

These are relatively uncommon as presenting problems, perhaps again because they may be subsumed under another heading, such as erectile failure. They can involve avoiding touching the partner's genitals or parts of the genitals such as the foreskin, or the avoidance of sexual feelings altogether. Whatever the exact nature of the problem, such reactions indicate a person in extreme distress, similar to a panic reaction, which leads them to go to great lengths to avoid the triggers to it (see Kaplan 1987).

Pain

Pain associated with sexual activity can occur for men in a number of ways. Sometimes there is generalized pain in the genital area, whereas in other cases it occurs when the man gets an erection, on ejaculation or following intercourse. Causes of such pain include problems with the foreskin and physical illnesses, such as a local infection. It can be a result of sexual activity itself when there is lack of lubrication, lack of ejaculation, or simply too much sex! Sometimes it has a psychological origin, such as where intense sexual feelings are interpreted as pain. There is also a significant group of male clients for whom no identifiable cause for the pain can be found.

Sexual problems manifesting primarily in a relationship

Differences of interest in sex

This can be characterized as a *relational* problem since it might not arise with a different partner having a similar level of sexual interest. As differences in levels of sexual interest between partners are common, in many cases a key element may be an inability to compromise. The problem can be fuelled by unrealistic expectations and be made worse by inflexibility, for example where one or both partners will not consider accepting relief of sexual tensions through masturbation as part of the way of managing the problem. It most commonly presents as the man being more interested in sex than the woman, but the extent of male lack of interest may be hidden by the cultural unacceptability of men expressing this. The options in dealing with this problem are to facilitate an increase of interest in one partner, a decrease of interest in the other, or to bring about some kind of compromise.

Difficulties in communicating about sex

Difficulty in communicating about sex may be part of a more general communication problem, although many couples who communicate well over other issues cannot do so over sex. It is common for couples to assume that they know each other's sexual needs and preferences. Many people think that communication about sexual practice is somehow abnormal or undesirable. As a result many people put up with practices that they do not enjoy, or do not say what they want sexually, while at the same time allowing their partner to assume that they are perfectly happy with what is happening.

A general relationship difficulty causing a sexual problem

Sexual problems are a common consequence of couple relationship problems. In order to engage in a sexual relationship most people need to be able to be vulnerable without feeling unsafe. This is not possible if significant degrees of anger, resentment or hostility are present in the relationship. On the other hand a relationship problem can be secondary to a sexual problem. It is difficult for many relationships to contain a sexual problem for a long time without it affecting other areas of the relationship. Thus sexual problems often lead to rows, misunderstandings, guilt, withdrawal and resentment.

The incidence and origins of sexual problems

It is notoriously difficult to obtain reliable general population data on sexual activity and practices. In conducting surveys there are obstacles to identifying a representative population, and it is hard to obtain a high response rate. Additionally there are all kinds of factors, such as embarrassment or bragging, that lead people to give false reports, to deny, to exaggerate or to give answers that they think the questioner will perceive as 'normal'. As regards the incidence of sexual problems some have gone so far as to suggest that the incidences of clinical sexual problems in the clinical and general populations are very close and that some sexual difficulty exists in most relationships. The issue then becomes why some present asking for help and others do not. In any event it is clear that the incidence of problems is huge compared with the numbers requesting treatment. Important issues in determining whether help is requested include the quality of the general relationship, the degree of importance of sexuality and sex to the individual or the couple, and the degree of sexual dissatisfaction as opposed to sexual dysfunction. Cultural and individual perceptions of how problems should be dealt with are also relevant. The perceived and actual availability of specialist services for sexual problems is also crucial.

In considering how sexual problems are generated it is easy to give plausible explanations, but it is rather more difficult to provide convincing proof. There are no standards for sexual behaviour or for the incidence of sexual problems in the general population. Moreover, we have no idea how factors we label as predisposing are distributed, and little idea about the characteristics of those who have sexual problems but do not present for help. We also have to be careful not to find problems where clients believe there to be none, and not to dismiss problems when clients experience them.

Classification of causes

A useful way of describing the causes of sexual problems is to categorize them as predisposing, precipitating or maintaining. Some predisposing factors make people vulnerable to a sexual difficulty but the problem does not emerge until a much later date. A precipitant factor is one that actually triggers the problem, and is the kind of causal factor the client is most likely to be aware of. Maintaining factors perpetuate the problem, sometimes in the absence of whatever triggered it in the first place. Some factors can operate in more than one way.

For example, anxiety can operate as a predisposing, precipitating and maintaining factor. If someone has a generally high anxiety level, a tendency to worry about problems, or a tendency to worry specifically about sex, this can make the person very vulnerable to a sexual difficulty. It is common for a period of anxiety or stress to trigger the emergence of a sexual difficulty. As a maintaining factor, anxiety operates mainly via performance anxiety, anticipation of failure, or spectatoring. In fact, anxiety is the state of mind most commonly linked with sexual problems. It interferes with the mental state required for sexual response and is disruptive of the ability to focus on sexual thoughts and sensations. Additionally it interferes with physical arousal by disrupting the response of the sympathetic nervous system. Paradoxically, though, sexual activity may increase if the anxiety is minor and not connected with sex!

Table 2.3 Classification of causes

Main predisposing factors
- restrictive upbringing – attitudes to sexuality and nudity; sex as wrong, dirty, evil
- lack of education – sexual myths, no education
- disturbed family relationships – lack of intimacy; no opportunity for modelling
- traumatic early sexual experiences – incest; rape – especially women

Main precipitant events
- childbirth leading to lack of interest by women and adjustments in the couple's relationship
- a long gap in lovemaking, the completion of the family, difficult pregnancy/birth
- discord in the general relationship – infidelity
- random failure
- ageing – performance change; worries over loss of attractiveness
- depression – part of the general loss of interest and the lack of desire to relate to others

Main maintaining factors
- performance anxiety, anticipation of failure, spectatoring
- guilt – about not responding; about being sexually needy
- poor communication
- discord in the relationship
- poor self-image – psychological or physical
- poor adaptation skills – inability to compromise, to negotiate, to change to accommodate new circumstances
- various detrimental circumstances – lack of privacy; lack of comfort; pressure of work; redundancy threat; unemployment

---

Atypical sexual behaviour

The varieties of sexual behaviours in which people engage are myriad, though the most common sexual fantasies and activity, such as penetrative sex and masturbation, focus on a limited range of desires and behaviours. Although many behaviours and fantasies do not fall into this general range, this does not necessarily mean that they are abnormal but, rather, may be considered atypical, reflecting the fact that the majority of people do not engage in them. Atypical sexual preferences often become defined as a problem by the person engaging in them when a need arises to change these behaviours but it is not possible to do so. Triggers to a wish for such change include incompatibility with a current relationship, actual or potential problems with the law and the desire to be 'normal'. Problematic atypical sexual behaviours are often referred to as paraphilias, the most common of which are forms of fetishism and various sado-masochistic practices. A distinction needs to be made between those that are non-coercive, such as fetishism or transvestism, and those that are coercive, such as voyeurism or sado-masochism.

Some of these, in a minor way, form part of many people's sexual repertoires, but here we are referring to situations where they take the form of impulsive or compulsive behaviours necessary for sexual arousal, and which cause difficulty and distress if the individual tries to stop them. Most commonly they present in men rather than women (see Gudjonsson 1986). In reality the difference between atypical and paraphiliac behaviour is often in degree rather than kind. Many men find that certain objects, such as stockings and suspenders, intensify their sexual arousal. For others it is a necessity for arousal, and the purpose of sex can become to have contact with such lingerie, and in such a case the behaviour would be considered paraphiliac. It is important to recognize that sexual orientation is not related to paraphilia, so that a gay exhibitionist, for example, is considered paraphiliac not because he is gay but because he exposes his genitals (Levin *et al.* 1990).

Gender problems present in a variety of ways and to differing degrees, ranging from people who have anxieties about their masculinity or femininity, to others whose genitalia and identity as men or women are discordant. In the later case distress is caused by the individual feeling trapped in the body of the wrong sex. This is known as gender dysphoria, and people experiencing this are known as transsexuals. Some wish to have hormonal and surgical treatments to re-assign their gender and often find sex dissatisfying until they have the anatomy of the desired gender. People often confuse transsexualism with cross-dressing and transvestism, but transvestites are clear about their gender identity and do not want to change this. Sometimes transsexualism and transvestism are confused with homosexuality and lesbianism. It is important to distinguish both from issues of sexual preference.

Problems about sexual orientation usually present as confusion about sexual identity; careful and sensitive exploration and assessment are needed to reveal the nature and extent of the problems. The traditional pathologizing of homosexuality in society can lead people to be fairly circumspect about raising such concerns, for fear of being labelled abnormal, or discovering something about themselves that may disrupt their lives. The resolution of worries about sexual orientation is important in enabling the individual to feel integrated and sexually fulfilled. It is worth remembering that, despite some societal changes, in Western culture heterosexuality is currently the only sexual orientation receiving full social legitimacy.

Some comments on normality

There are difficulties in deciding what might be considered a sexual *problem* and what is to be thought of as *normal*. A statistical definition might be appealing, defining the average and the normal range, but we have already seen how difficult it is to establish any reliable norms. An obvious solution might be to let clients define both their problems and the desired outcomes, but this could be unrealistic if, for instance, what the client wants is physiologically impossible! Arguments from physiology about what is normal tend to focus on reproductive function and do not take sufficient account of individual differences, cultural factors or possible limitations in our physiological knowledge. Guidelines from social norms are difficult because values and expectations shift, and in any case vary between different cultures and groups. The danger in such a definition of normality is that it is arbitrary and does not reflect the diversity of people's background and experience.

It could also be argued that cultural norms about sexuality are overly influenced by certain sectors of society, in particular the media and professionals. Women's magazines, newspapers, the cinema, television and videos exert a powerful influence through their sexual imagery. The implicit and explicit values which they promote can shape beliefs and expectations. Professionals can also have a disproportionate influence, including agony aunts, GPs, gynaecologists and therapists. Similarly difficulties attend arguments about normality derived from religion and ethics.

We therefore need to take care in making any sweeping statements about normality. Counsellors and therapists must be vigilant in order to avoid imposing their own values and desired outcomes on clients. In thinking about the goals of therapy, account must obviously be taken of a number of aspects, particularly physiology, social norms and belief systems. In this way it should be possible to ensure that people are not aiming for the physiologically impossible, that they are not left with an unbearable tension with their own or surrounding social norms, and that they are helped to sort out their sexuality within the context of their particular ethical and religious beliefs.

Cultural and ethnic differences

It is inevitable that the various forms of psychological help reflect and transmit the values of the prevailing culture, and for this reason understanding cultural bias is important (see Holmes 1996). Counselling and psychotherapy are not value free, and we need to be able to analyse our own countertransference reactions and how these influence our practice. This should lead to the creation of a sensitive and culturally relevant psychodynamic approach that can contain sexual symptomology and the associated psychological distress. Part of this means being aware of how our own value system conflicts with or supports our clients' values.

The way that sexual problems are classified assumes certain values about the place of sex, leading to the construction of a particular model of sexuality that may largely reflect Western middle-class life and not take sufficient account of cultural diversity (Daines 1988). There has been little research on ethnicity and sexual problems, but as Lavee (1991) notes, the dominant Western model makes four assumptions about sexuality:

- Sex is primarily a means of exchanging pleasure.
- Both partners are equally involved.
- People need and want information about sex.
- Communication is important for good sexual relationships.

These assumption are not generalizable to other non-Western groups and cultures. When working with Arab, North African, and Asian Jews in Israel, Lavee found that most of his clients were men with erectile difficulties. Some complained of premature ejaculation, but only when it interfered with their own pleasure. There was no appreciation of how this problem affected the partner, and often the man would attend for therapy alone.

The usual cognitive-behavioural approach was resisted, and most clients dropped out of the therapy.

The eroticization of Western contemporary culture through sexual symbolism and acting out has been marked in recent decades, and sometimes it can seem that sex is all-pervasive. It is routinely used to sell consumer products; it has caused the downfall of public figures from politicians to clergy; it has contributed towards a climate in which the pursuit of peak sexual experiences is often seen as some kind of ultimate answer in life. Horrocks (1997) calls this 'neurotic eroticization' and believes that it is designed to avoid the deep sense of abandonment and deprivation that people feel who engage in sex addictively. This reverses Freud's understanding of the relationship between sexuality and human motivation. Horrocks states 'it throws doubt on his claim that neurosis has a sexual aetiology. Rather, one could argue that neurosis has a sexual expression! Sex is a great aspirin or tranquilliser for many people' (Horrocks 1997: 124).

There are many issues to be considered when working with people from different cultural and ethnic groups. Firstly there are different cultural definitions of what constitutes a problem. If the purpose of sex is defined as male pleasure or the need to produce children, then some of the problems that women experience, such as lack of orgasm or low sexual desire, do not become issues to be addressed unless they interfere with intercourse. Other problems such as vaginismus or painful intercourse are likely to have a direct effect on a woman's ability to have intercourse, and consequently may be more likely to be perceived as a problem.

The ways in which these problems will become defined, though, will be consistent with the belief system of a culture where sex is not for female pleasure but for reproduction and male pleasure. It is not easy to know whether women in such cultures perceive sex solely in this way, because of difficulties associated with women speaking out, especially on such personal and private issues. D'Ardenne and Mahtani (1989) suggest that we try to listen to our clients' cultural norms and try to keep our own values out of the process. Becoming sensitive to such issues enables us to work across cultures with client groups who have been traditionally marginalized. More debate and research is needed within sex therapy about the potential contributions and problems that may arise out of the cultural aspects and implications of a specifically psychodynamic approach.

Explanations of causes

While religion nowadays has less impact on many people's lives in Britain, for some groups this is still a major factor to consider in their treatment. For example, certain clients may have objections to practices that form part of the treatment processes in sex therapy, such as masturbation. Others may have either cultural or religious objections to an approach that does not offer the hope of penetrative sex. Some religious beliefs encompass a whole world-view in which reliance on science and scientific thinking does not sit comfortably. It has become increasingly recognized that the pursuit of science implies certain values. Facts do not exist in a vacuum but within the context of assumptions that are determined by particular values, and it is not to be assumed that these values are superior to the alternatives. An interesting challenge to traditional Western assumptions is discussed by Horton (1967), who addresses the differences between African traditional thought and Western science. He shows how Western medical remedies may be less effective than African traditional ones in certain situations, because the latter indirectly recognize the role of social disturbance in the causation of some illnesses. Most sex therapists recognize the ineffectiveness of mainstream sex therapy with certain client groups, largely because they are working within scientific assumptions that are not shared by the clients.

> With his wife, Emma, Craig attended complaining of an erectile problem which, on taking a full history, seemed to be related to his diabetes. This was explained to them together with the kind of help that might rectify the problem. They were told that they had to be prepared for the eventuality that the outcome might be restricted to assisting them to find ways of making love that did not depend on penetration. However, both were adamant that they were not interested in this. For them, they said, love-making involved intercourse, and if this turned out not to be possible, then they would rather not engage in sexual activity at all.

> Fred and June, a couple in their sixties, seemed initially willing to attempt to adjust to the limitations of Fred's lack of erection. However, as time went on it became clear that they were unable to see this as anything other than a

very inadequate substitute for what they wanted. Their religious beliefs led them to see a great qualitative difference between intercourse and other lovemaking activities. Eventually they chose to discontinue sexual contact.

There are also important cultural differences about where it is seen as appropriate to take problems. In Latin America problems are often thought to be caused by supernatural forces, and so healers are called in to bring charms and medicines to ward off evil spirits. In some cultures women can talk among their extended families but men are discouraged from discussing their problems, this being seen as a sign of weakness. Lavee concludes: 'If the client's sexual values are different, we ought to remember that a well integrated life philosophy, that has proven effective for generations, stands behind them. It may therefore be easier and wiser to fit the treatment to the client's values than to attempt to "teach" them what healthy sex is' (Lavee 1991: 212).

The conjunction of sexual and couple relationship problems

Sexual problems often present in the context of a relationship, whether a lifelong partnership or one involving a more limited commitment. Scharff and Scharff (1991: 27) say that 'a poor sexual relationship is most often a product of object relations difficulty'. Additionally a good-enough sexual life 'supports the overall relatedness of a couple, providing solace and holding for domestic strain, and offers pleasurable regeneration of the couple's loving bond. Absence of sex has the opposite effect, aggravating the wear and tear, spreading frustration and a sense of rejection, and undermining the maintenance of the bond.' Even individuals presenting for help who do not have a partner usually have ideas or fantasies about a future relationship, which are often a relevant consideration in helping them. The complex interaction between relationships and sexual functioning means that clients and professionals may come to differing views in their assessment of whether the sexual problem or relationship difficulty is primary.

Polonsky and Nadelson (1982) point out how couples often present with a sexual problem, only for a relationship difficulty to emerge. Similarly couples who present with relationship problems sometimes have an associated sexual problem. Whatever the presenting problem, counsellors and psychotherapists need to be able to conduct a broad assessment of the relative influence of various factors. It is important to realize that there is never a purely physical sexual problem, as even the most obviously organic conditions (e.g. erectile failure due to nerve damage resulting from a prostate operation) often have a psychological element. Additionally, all problems have psychological consequences and most have repercussions for couple relationships. Part of the reason that sexual difficulties present as a distinct treatment category is because clients tend to see their sexual functioning in an overly physical way, and this influences how they present their problems. For the clinician, one of the distinctive elements of this kind of work is that, for some dysfunctions, the use of physical treatments or physical techniques alongside psychotherapy may be needed to produce the outcome desired by clients.

Conclusion

A psychodynamic understanding of sexual difficulties offers an approach that can take account of the many different roots of the problems that have been considered in this chapter. Understanding the interaction of the biological, emotional, sexual, cultural and relational factors enables the therapist to use a holistic understanding of the ways that sexual difficulties occur and persist. From this understanding, psychodynamic interventions can be made that take account of the multiplicity of factors that affect sexual function. As the next chapter makes clear, central to the psychodynamic approach is an understanding of the unconscious, and a belief that there are elements to people's behaviour in addition to those that appear on the surface. Within the context of sexual difficulties a psychodynamic approach offers a perspective that helps counter the splits between the mind and body that occur within so much of medicine and psychotherapy. Clearly sexual function itself straddles this split, and psychodynamic counselling and psychotherapy needs to be able to contain both the physical and the psychological aspects. In the following chapter we look in more detail at the relevant psychodynamic theory, and from this we develop a psychodynamic approach to sexuality and sexual problems, out of which the more practical issues of psychodynamic assessment and therapy are developed.

Chapter 3

Psychodynamic foundations: psychoanalysis, object relations and couple relationships

Origins in psychoanalysis

In trying to define what constitutes psychodynamic psycho-therapy or counselling it is helpful to set the term in its historical context. Its foundations lie in the theories of Freud from which the many developments in psychoanalytic theory and practice have followed. Originally Freud was concerned with producing an investigative model to understand the human mind and the influence of early experiences on psychological development, and in the development of his techniques of analysis. His studies involved the nature of neurotic difficulties, how symptoms arise, and exploring the role of the unconscious. He was concerned less about practical applications and more about developing the science of psycho-analysis (Freud 1933: 192).

Freud's model of psychological development is underpinned by an emphasis on biological drives and instincts, and the ways in which these come into conflict with aspects of the personality and with the external world. In particular he emphasized the role played by the sex drive in motivating peoples' behaviour. The psyche and the personality are in constant struggle with these instincts and drives in their search for expression and gratification. In this theory of drives other people are significant in the sense that they either help or hinder the individual in pursuit of the satisfaction of these drives. The personality is seen as a battlefield with central themes of division and conflict, and internal tension and adaption. The degree of conflict is mediated by the use of defence mechanisms which ensure that incompatible wishes remain unconscious or hidden, the main one of these being repression. For Freud the origins of all psychological illness can be traced back to the childhood experiences remaining repressed in the unconscious mind. There is an intrinsic tendency for these repressed wishes and impulses to return to consciousness, and so tension of one kind or another is therefore an inevitable and innate part of the system.

In developing his theory of mind Freud moved through three major phases, starting with the effect the environment has on the psyche, through to intrapsychic factors, and finally an increasing acknowledgement of the relationship between the two. He stated that neuroses derive from the 'incompatibility of the demands of civilisation and those of the instincts, and the tension between the desire to love and be loved by one's parents, and the fear of inevitable rivalry and the consequences this arouses' (Bateman and Holmes 1995: 5). Freud believed that the demands of society are in inevitable opposition to the individual's needs and, as the individual is dependent upon the wider group, repression and neuroses become the price the individual has to pay to fit into society.

Defining 'psychodynamic'

Psychoanalytic theory has been the major influence on the development of psychotherapy and counselling during the twentieth century. Many approaches have evolved from Freud's classical model, including many that have arisen out of a direct rejection of psychoanalysis. The proliferation of counselling and psychotherapy has led to a process of formalization of these into professions with formal registration and accredited trainings. The need to demonstrate value for money and cost-effectiveness in the NHS has led to the need to prove effectiveness of outcome for all forms of psychological help. In these contexts it has become necessary to clearly define terms such as 'psychoanalytic' and 'psychodynamic'. The problems of definition are further complicated by the research evidence indicating that it is not easy to determine which theoretical school a psychotherapist belongs to simply from a description of their activity (Heine 1953; Maguire 1973). One reason for this is that the term 'psychodynamic' may be used by practitioners to mean differing things.

Additionally there are a number of factions within psychoanalysis that seek exclusive use of psychoanalytic theory and terminology. An association with the practice of psychodynamic psychotherapy is seen by them as a dilution of psychoanalytic practice and as such is not supported. The limitations and constraints of belonging to only one 'school' are stultifying, as seen in the problems associated with the issue of the registration of psychotherapists, reflected in the tensions between the UK Council for Psychotherapy and the British Confederation of Psychotherapists (see Balfour and Richards 1995; Gardner 1995; Pokorny 1995).

Psychoanalysis itself has taken various directions in different countries as it has been subject to diverse social, cultural and political forces. Research evidence has repeatedly suggested that it is the qualities in the psychotherapeutic relationship that are important rather than diagnosis and technique (Fiedler 1950; Norcross 1977; Clarkson 1990). It has been found that differing kinds of relationship are needed for different kinds of clients, and this factor is most important when predicting the effectiveness of psychotherapy (Norcross 1997). This should be considered in the practice of psychosexual therapy in relation to the wide range of difficulties that clients bring.

Historically the term 'psychodynamic' does not appear in Freud's work, yet various authors have pointed to Freud's use of dynamic imagery in his work. For example when Freud is describing his theory of neurosis he uses the image of repressed, blocked off energy that seeks expression. He also uses the illustration of dammed up water to express the conflictual forces that a person struggles with both unconsciously and consciously, the person's symptoms being the conscious manifestation of this struggle. Rycroft (1972: 38) points out that psychoanalysis has a psychodynamic view of human development. He suggests that the difference is that psychoanalysis describes a method of psychotherapy and an overall theory of human development whereas 'psychodynamic' is a type of psychology. As with other types of psychology, such as behavioural or systems, the psychodynamic approach has developed into a form of psychotherapy drawing on a number of related theoretical works.

For Lidmilla (1996) the practice of what is called psychodynamic psychotherapy varies, and the term is used in ambiguous and confused ways to the extent that he sees a need to clarify the term. He distinguishes four separate ways in which 'psychodynamic' is currently being used to describe therapeutic activity

(Lidmilla 1996: 436). Two of the four definitions are pertinent to our current concerns:

- psychodynamic psychotherapy as an applied, probably modified, psychoanalytic practice;
- psychodynamics as a superordinate meta-psychology, with variable applications and practices, all of which show a common epistemology.

Both these definitions are relevant to our purpose in defining psychodynamic sex therapy. Jacobs suggests that in practice the psychodynamic approach is more flexible because it

> embraces the different psychoanalytic views on the structure of personality, by emphasizing the dynamic more than the structure. It allows for different models of developmental stages as well as gender and societal issues, all contributing more dynamic dimensions to our understanding of how the psyche forms and functions.
>
> (Jacobs 1994: 90)

For Jacobs the distinctiveness of the term 'psychodynamic' is to be found in its attention to the *process* – the way or manner – in which the personality develops and interacts with others.

In terms of our approach in this book we define 'psychodynamic' as an approach to psychotherapy or counselling whose theoretical model rests on a psychoanalytic understanding of the structure of the mind and its influences. These are seen in the conscious ways that people relate and express themselves but are also in the unconscious, from where they can be accessed and made conscious through interpretation. We address the way that mental processes function and are managed from this perspective. The emphasis is on the dynamic way in which the structure of the mind functions, the interrelationship with conscious and unconscious activities within the self, and the dynamic relationship that exists between the individual, significant others and wider society.

The aim in our approach is not analysis, though an analytic attitude by the therapist is often necessary whereby language and meaning are emphasized, and active problem-solving interventions by the therapist are discouraged. The overriding focus is not on the style and technique upon which analysts place so much importance, but on how the relationship between therapist and client generates the dynamics that are contained and worked upon in the sessions. Working with the unconscious and developing the transference are important, and the use of insight and interpretation are essential. However, the nature of the work may be also shaped by a number of other factors, such as the nature of the presenting problem, the setting and the client's own agenda. Such psychodynamic psychotherapy and counselling can be offered in a number of different modalities – individual or couple, short or long term in duration – and with a flexibility that allows its inclusion as part of a multidisciplinary team approach that includes a variety of therapeutic ways of working.

Approaching sexual difficulties psychodynamically

Working psychodynamically with sexual difficulties places an emphasis on the dynamic aspects of difficulties in an area of life which is influenced by a number of complex, interrelated factors, such as physical and mental health, societal expectations, and ideas about normal sexual practice. There are aspects of Freudian theory that still influence our understanding of sexuality and sexual functioning, but the theoretical underpinning of our approach relies particularly on modern developments in contemporary psychoanalytic theory which relate to unconscious motivations and explanations for partner choice and sexual difficulties. These broaden out, and in some instances supersede, Freud's ideas of sexual drives, impulses, stages and erotic zones. The major shift is towards the importance of others in our psychological development. This move away from drive theory towards what is called object relations has carried with it a change in emphasis on sexuality, which has become less central in the construction of theories of personality development. The making and sustaining of personal relationships and their effects on the individual have come more into focus. However, in tracing these developments in more detail, it is with Freud's ideas that we need to begin.

Freud on psychosexual development

Around the end of the nineteenth century Freud first published his theories about sexuality, which were revised and refined over the next twenty or more years. His understanding shifted from the biologism of drive theory to a model of sexuality concerned with the 'sexual object', in particular the triangular relationship expressed in terms of the Oedipus complex. From this Freud was able to develop an overall theory of psychosexual development within which libido represents the biological sexual energy underpinning the development of the personality and the ability of the individual to form relationships. For Freud the term 'libido' meant a form of sexual energy, but since then it has taken on an indiscriminate sexual meaning.

Freud broke new ground in his recognition of the sexual instinct in the infant, publishing his initial theory and observations in the 'Three essays on the theory of sexuality' (1905: 33–155). At the time Freud's revelations of erotic impulses and fantasies in early childhood caused great controversy. Freud believed that these sexual thoughts and feelings are part and parcel of the unfolding psychological development of the normal child. He used the case study of a 5-year-old boy – little Hans – to show the infantile Oedipal conflicts behind his phobic symptoms (1909: 165–317). The combination of instinctual drives, impulses and Oedipal fantasies results in the conscious mind needing to defend itself against unconscious incestuous wishes. In the 'little Hans' case the little boy's feelings and thoughts had become attached to another object – horses – as he became preoccupied with them and the size of their genitals. Freud interpreted these symptoms in the light of Hans's incestuous wishes towards his mother, his death wish towards his father, and his fear of his father's retaliatory anger. He believed that Hans was defending himself from these primitive feelings through his symptoms. His fear of horses was therefore a sophisticated evasion, a way of coping with emotions which he dare not freely admit to himself. Freud saw this case as illustrating a route to uncovering the basis of neuroses occurring in adult life:

> The physician who treats an adult psychoanalytically, at last reaches through his work of uncovering psychical formations, layer by layer, certain hypotheses about infantile sexuality in whose components he believes he has found the motive forces of all neurotic symptoms of later life.
>
> (Freud 1909: 169–70)

The healthy resolution of the Oedipal conflict involves a boy's identification with his father, and repression and sublimation of incestuous wishes. The latter means giving up hope of possessing his mother sexually, thus symbolically castrating himself. Identification with his father leads him to introject – to take inside himself – the paternal prohibition of sexuality and aggression. Thus the father becomes part of the son, and society's mores are accepted. At the same time the boy has to preserve enough acceptance of his own sexual potency to be able to achieve extra-familial sexual relationships in adulthood. Freud's theories of sexual development include the now familiar oral, anal and genital stages, associated with a preoccupation with, and gratification from, corresponding erotogenic zones. In later childhood the latency period is entered. Karl Abraham elaborated on the earlier stages and created subdivisions, such as anal retentive and anal expulsive (Abraham 1924). Erikson's developmental model adds various stages covering adulthood and old age (Erikson 1965: ch. 7).

As the main sexual object for a child is his or her own body, one of the main features of infantile sexual life is auto-eroticism, dominated by the urge for instant gratification. The baby seeks gratification from her own body, or from her mother's body, which is barely differentiated from the baby's own. This infantile sexual behaviour has polymorphous aims, and in this sense Freud saw perversion as a normal part of sexual development. Adult neurotic sexuality, for example, is seen as a regression to an infantile state. He argues that if normal sexual development is repressed for some reason, then the sexual instinct flows into ancillary channels formed from the components of the ever-changing aims of the infantile sexuality.

Thus Freud connects sexual development from childhood to the origin of neuroses and perversions that occur in adults. The key aspect for Freud is the impact of constitutional, as opposed to environmental, influences on a person's sexual development. So, for example, when discussing perversions he makes his famous statement that we are all perverse, since perversion is innate in everyone, although it varies in its intensity and may be increased by events in a person's life (Freud 1905: 87). However, he does not explore this in any detail, but goes on to explore how the innate roots of this instinct grow into expressions of sexual activity in some, while in others they are repressed and become symptoms in psychoneuroses.

Puberty for Freud heralds the sexual instinct in pursuit of objects, not in a relational sense, but as an independent biological process quite separate from relationships. In adulthood, the 'normal sexual aim is regarded as being the union of genitals in the act known as copulation, which leads to the release of the sexual tension and a temporary extinction of the sexual instinct' (Freud 1905: 61). On the question of object choice, this may not necessarily be a person of the opposite sex; in fact Freud considered bisexuality to be a part of normal development and a component of every person's sexuality. Additionally Young (1996) points out that although Freud thought homosexuality could be a developmental inhibition, he did not regard it as a perversion or illness. He also thought it could be innate, or triggered by certain environmental conditions (e.g. prison).

Freud on the psychosexual development of girls

Freud assumes that the psychosexual world of girls is somewhat similar to that of boys. They also wish to replace their same-sex parent in order to win the opposite-sex parent, in this case the all-powerful father. Unlike boys, however, girls associate their lack of a penis with feeling powerless and insignificant. From this Freud hypothesizes that women dislike masturbation as it is a masculine activity. He believes that a woman cannot cope with this pleasurable activity because it gives her a 'narcissistic sense of humiliation which is bound up with penis-envy, the remainder that after all she cannot compete with boys and that it would therefore be best for her to give up the idea of doing so' (Freud 1925: 340). However, Freud's view is that the girl does not totally give up her feelings towards her father in the same way that boys do with their mother; rather, a girl 'gives up her wish for a penis and puts in place of it a wish for a child and *with that purpose in view* she takes her father as love object' (p. 340, emphasis in original).

True resolution of the Oedipus complex for the girl is therefore not possible, as the fantasy of possessing the father is carried on through marriage and the birth of her own male child, the possessor and symbol of the missing penis. Fisher (1993: 147–8) concludes that 'Freud's solution in reference to the little girl was to develop a convoluted, changing account of her Oedipus complex.' Freud (1925: 323–4) himself came to the conclusion that in girls the motive for the demolition of the Oedipus complex is lacking, and so its effects may persist far into women's normal mental life. 'Their super-ego is never so exorable, so impersonal, so independent of its emotional origins as we require it to be in men' (Freud 1925: 324).

Freud's view of female arousal and orgasm

Despite the shortcomings in Freud's views on female psycho-sexual development, they were influential at the time and have continued to resonate. Freud's phallocentric view of women's sexuality led him to postulate that women not only desperately desire a penis, but that physically the clitoris is a homologue of the penis. This later paved the way for him to characterize the clitoral sexuality of the little girl as 'masculine'. 'The leading erotogenic zone in female children is located at the clitoris, and is thus homologous to the masculine genital zone of the glans penis' (Freud 1905: 142). He describes the clitoris as the initial sexual zone and uses an image of kindling to describe its sexual role:

> When at last the sexual act is permitted and the clitoris itself becomes excited, it still retains a function: namely, of trans-mitting the excitation to the adjacent female sexual parts, just as . . . pine shavings can be kindled in order to set a log of harder wood on fire.

> (p. 143)

He goes on to suggest that for a girl to become a woman sexually she has eventually to transfer the main erotic zone from the clitoris to the vagina. 'The process of the girl becoming a woman depends very much on the clitoris passing on this sensitivity to the vaginal orifice in good time and completely' (pp. 143–4).

Freud believes that females accomplish the task of this trans-fer of zones at puberty, a transfer in which the clitoral zone must entirely renounce its sensitivity. This change finds no parallel in the development of males. He is vague and inconsistent about its timing, postulating that it occurs at the phallic stage (age 4 to 5 years) in some writings, and in others at a later time. However, he does point out that other factors may affect female orgasmic function and dysfunction, as when he writes about 'anaesthesia'. Here he suggests that psychic determinants play a part, as also do zones other than the vagina and the clitoris:

> Anaesthesia in women, as is well known, is often only apparent and local. They are anaesthetic at the vaginal orifice but are by no means incapable of excitement origi-nating in the clitoris or even in other zones. Alongside these erotogenic determinants of anaesthesia must also be set the psychical determinants, which arise from repression.

> (p. 143)

This concept of vaginal anaesthesia is caused in part by repression of the libido, but what is unclear is his view of the erotogenic determinants of the anaesthesia, or what other zones explicitly are involved in female arousal. More fundamentally it is not clear on what evidence Freud was basing the assertion that anaesthesia in women is well known. He raises more questions than answers, but at least gives the suggestion that women have other psychological and anatomic influences on their libido.

Freud's view of female sexuality, and in particular the nature of the female orgasm, is controversial, and special notoriety has surrounded his explanation of orgasmic problems. In particular the idea of the inferiority of the clitoral orgasm and the existence of a distinctive and 'mature' vaginal orgasm has been attributed to Freud. However, it is important to point out that he never once in his writings characterizes clitoral or vaginal orgasms as separate entities, or in fact ever uses the term 'orgasm'. Therefore the clitoral versus vaginal orgasm debate is founded more on inferences from Freud, than on what he actually said. What is apparent is that Freud has great difficulty providing a clear and consistent account of female psychosexual development, and acknowledges this difficulty. He admits to not fully understanding females when he famously states that 'We know less about the sexual life of little girls than of boys. But we need not feel ashamed of this distinction; after all, the sexual life of adult women is a "dark continent" for psychology' (p. 63).

Freud has been heavily criticized for his inadequate and male centred view of female sexual development. For example, women *do* have vaginal sensation, and clitoral arousal is not transitory, but an integral and enduring part of the physiological response. Perhaps the overriding difficulty is that his explanation sees female sexuality as derivative from the male:

> Freud consistently argued that the little girl is biologically masculine. In a sense, female sexuality does not exist in its own right until the shock of the castration complex forces girls to abandon masculinity and seek femininity – since she cannot have a penis for herself, she must try to receive one from a man.
>
> (Horrocks 1997: 60)

Freud's understanding of sexual symptoms

For Freud the specific and sole causes of sexual pathology are unresolved Oedipal problems, both for men and women. A

Freudian formulation of women's sexual difficulties, for example, rests on the central issue of unresolved penis envy, which Freud believes underlies women's psychological difficulties generally. Thus vaginismus can be seen as a hysterical or conversion symptom, a symbolic expression of psychic conflict where envy and hostility to men exists because of penis envy. Orgasmic difficulties arise where penis envy impedes a transition from the clitoris to the vagina, and can lead to no orgasm at all (Kaplan 1974: 166–82). Similarly for men, sexual problems such as erectile difficulties can be understood in terms of castration anxiety – anxiety about acting out incestuous feelings and desires and incurring the retaliatory fear of his father lead to unresolvable internal tension and conflict, which in turn precludes effective sexual functioning.

Freud was particularly interested in understanding the psychology of male impotence. In 'On the universal tendency to debasement in the sphere of love', he gives his most explicit account. He states that the inability to form a normal attitude in love is because 'two currents . . . have failed to combine' (Freud 1912: 248). Affection and sensuality are not linked, but rather opposed as a result of incestuous fantasies which evoke castration fears as the man tries to make love. The capacity to love becomes marked by this split, and the man finds 'restriction has thus been placed on the object choice' (Freud 1910: 232). Freud discusses these restrictions in terms of a split between affection for the idealized, 'instinctual mother', and sensuality towards the debased prostitute-like surrogate woman. This product of the Oedipal dynamics represents a form of immaturity, specifically a developmental failure to be able to direct sexual desire and love towards the same object.

> Carole and Ken presented asking for help with Ken's erectile problems. They had met when Carole had gone to her insurance brokers to report the theft of her car; Ken was the insurance broker who took her details. Carole worked as a table-top dancer in a local nightclub. They both described finding each other very sexually attractive and, prior to living together, their sexual life was fulfilling. However, since living together their sexual interest in each other had deteriorated, and it emerged that Ken's erectile difficulties were secondary to his loss of sexual interest. During this time Carole had given up her erotic dancing and spent more time at home, especially

to support Ken, who had been experiencing pressure at work.

When they were both asked about their feelings about these changes they both expressed relief about Carole stopping work, together with disgust at the men who go to such places and the women who work there. They denied that it formed part of any attraction between them, and supported this by pointing out that Ken had never visited Carole in her place of work. However, as therapy progressed, it did emerge that Ken had fantasized about Carole in her work, though Carole denied that the erotic dancing was in any way sexual to her or that she enjoyed the attentiveness of the customers. It was as if the erotic aspects of their life together had been separated from the maternal aspects, and they were both fearful to hold both these parts of their relationship together. Ken's erectile difficulties prevented them combining the erotic and the maternal as his sexual fantasies consciously kept Carole the erotic dancer separate from Carole his partner. It is interesting that Carole remarked in one session that it was as if her life as a dancer was someone else and not her, and Ken agreed with this.

Their behaviours were protecting them from any incestuous anxieties, but proving unsatisfactory in meeting their needs to be close to each other. The anxiety was expressed in a fear that they would drift apart. Therapy progressed with both of them exploring the meanings of their attraction to each and the restrictions on their sexual life. In the course of this they discovered that they shared common feelings about erotic dancing which were connected with the tension between what was available and unavailable. This realization made the idea less sexually attractive. They were thus able to work through this, along with Carole's need to be maternal towards Ken.

Kaplan (1974: 328) further summarizes classical psychoanalytic understanding of other common psychosexual problems, such as premature ejaculation and non-ejaculation. For example, she suggests that premature ejaculation can be seen as expressing unconscious sadistic feelings towards women, soiling and defiling women, and depriving her of pleasure. Non-ejaculation can be understood as an expression of castration anxiety, the man believing that he will be injured or harmed in some way if he ejaculates into the vagina. These unconscious ambivalent feelings find symbolic expression in the symptom of 'ejaculatory incontinence' (p. 328).

Freud's legacy and object relations

Freud's 'Three essays on the theory of sexuality' represented a radical theoretical shift in the understanding of psychosexual development, and gave sexual development a central role in the formation of the personality. However, Freud's characterization of human beings as essentially passive within an autonomous biological process, brought the history of psychoanalytical thought into a cul-de-sac (Horrocks 1997: 49). Subsequent research and writing has moved away from biology towards interpersonal aspects. The beginning of this trend can be seen in the development of object-relations approaches by Klein, Fairbairn and Winnicott, which depart from classical libido theory. While there are important differences between them, they all brought to the fore an emphasis on relations with objects, rather than the expression of instincts. In this context, an object is to be understood as that to which desire or action is directed. Usually this will be a person, but it can be part of a person, such as the breast, or even a non-human symbol (Rycroft 1972: 100).

The crucial change is that libido no longer determines object relations, but rather that object relations determine libido (Greenberg and Mitchell 1983: 157). The main effects of object relations on psychoanalytic thinking was firstly to point to relations with the good and bad aspects of the mother and other important figures and part-objects; and secondly to treat relations with objects, rather than the expression of instincts, as the basic preoccupation of psychoanalytic thinking and clinical work. In this process the individual's psychic functioning is constellated through their interactions with others, and their psychosexual development is seen as secondary to these attachments. These external relationships with objects and part-objects are internalized, becoming 'internal objects' in the person's mind and relating to the central self and to each other.

Modern views of the Oedipus conflict

In this section we draw on Young's (1996) deliberations on the issue of perversion in relation to the Oedipus complex, although some of our conclusions are different. One problem with the framework as we have looked at it so far is its restriction to Oedipal themes to explain and understand sexual problems. The idea that the essential genesis of adult sexual problems lies only in infantile Oedipal conflicts is no longer widely accepted. Equally contentious is the assumption that the satisfactory resolution of the Oedipus conflict leads to heterosexuality, and that any other outcome implies continuing psychopathology. Many contemporary psychoanalytic writers have intensely debated these aspects of the Freudian model of psychosexual development, and have moved away from a literal acceptance to broad understanding of the themes or metaphors that are suggested by the Oedipus complex. Themes of intimacy and separation, of similarity and difference, are worked out in the three-person drama of two parents and the child. This offers the child an opportunity to develop boundaries and limits and to be able to contain envy, anger, separateness and closeness, without feeling abandoned, destroyed or overwhelmed. Analysts such as Klein shift the focus to the early relationship between the baby and the mother, and emphasize pre-Oedipal experiences, as we shall see later in our discussion.

The classical Freudian psychosexual schema generates criteria by which normal sexual and emotional developments are measured. Thus if someone misses out a stage, becomes stuck at any point, or misses out a developmental task, then perversion or even psychosis may follow. A pseudo-maturity is gained, whereby sexual interest and gratification are focused on a substitute object rather than the appropriate one. Such processes are seen as essentially neurotic, as are instances of sexual interest and gratification which are seen as outside the normal. At the other end of the spectrum there are theories that reject biology as the determining factor and see people as making choices about their sexuality. The beginning of this trend can be seen in the movement away from biology and drive theory in the development of object-relations approaches by Klein and Fairbairn.

Most object-relations theorists agree with Hiller (1996) that the Oedipus complex is resolved when the child recognizes and accepts the reality of exclusion from the parental sexual relationship. Acceptance of the link between the parents leads to the necessity of seeing oneself as capable of interactions outside the parents–child triangle. The child combines her parents' projections of themselves as a couple with her own perceptions, both accurate and projected. Once the focus is on relations rather than drives, sexuality and sexual energy no longer provide the conceptual framework for how we think about the inner world. Love, hatred, unconscious phantasy, anxiety and defences come to the foreground, as we shall see when we discuss Dicks's ideas below. Modern theories therefore offer more sophisticated and sensitive ways than traditional psychoanalytic theories of understanding sexual problems. They have their root in attempting to understand how couple relationships form and have their origins in early object relations.

An important aspect of the Kleinian view of the resolution of the Oedipus complex is that it involves the same elements as the depressive position: 'the two situations are inextricably intertwined in such a way that one cannot be resolved without the other: we resolve the Oedipus complex by working through the depressive position and the depressive position by working through the Oedipus complex' (Britton 1992: 35). Fisher (1993: 145) usefully outlines current Kleinian thought on the Oedipus complex in 'The impenetrable other: ambivalence and the Oedipal conflict in work with couples'. He says that the 'capacity to be an individual, to be separate and hence capable of a relationship with another, rests on mastering the anxieties of the triangle' (p. 145). The depressive position describes the situation where a child realizes that his love and hate are both directed towards the same object, the mother. Anxieties are raised about what damage may have been done by the hate and the child tries to make reparation for this and to work through his ambivalence.

There are also anxieties about being excluded from the couple relationship, and of being in a couple relationship that excludes the third person. The experience of ambivalence, in the form of the feelings of love and hate directed towards the same person, is intimately linked with these anxieties and their resolution. Whereas the resolving of these results in a sense of psychological space, failure to do so leads to a lack of any sense of psychological or emotional space. Such space is needed for a person to think for him or herself, to be able to be different and separate from others and to begin or end a relationship. Complete resolution is not possible as the anxieties 'are only ever resolved provisionally, *never finally*, and they are commonly, and sometimes even dramatically, revived in the intimacy of a couple relationship' (Fisher 1993: 145, emphasis in original). Therefore the 'Oedipal constellation' is something that recurs throughout life, especially in close relationships. It is not surprising, therefore, that it is an underlying feature of many of the problems for which couples seek help.

One of the strong arguments against the classical psycho-analytic position, whether Freudian or Kleinian, is that they fail to recognize that the division between the psychic and socio-political (including the existence of the Oedipus complex as an internal process) has itself arisen out of a particular discourse that is socially and culturally specific. Therefore the prescriptions arising from the classical psychoanalytic position come to be seen as resting on an illegitimate attempt to speak from beyond social and cultural influence. Once this is conceded, concerns about normality or perversion recede, to be replaced by issues connected with sexual preferences and choices. Clearly the impact of biology cannot be completely ignored, but its role in determining sexual matters is diminished. One of the consequences of this is that the boundary between the normal and the abnormal, or the normal and the perverse, does not exist in the same way. Therefore O'Connor and Ryan (1993) attack the views of many within psychoanalysis that lesbianism should be understood as, for example, a narcissistic condition or a defence against psychosis. Together with others (e.g. Ellis 1987) they draw on the ideas of Foucault to show the socio-historical specificity of lesbian and gay identities (Foucault 1984). Ellis (1987: 373) claims that 'psychoanalytic theory, while claiming to be value free and based on "observation" is instead a conflation of medical, legal and moral discourses'; and that it rests on the assumption that 'sexual identity can be viewed in isolation from social context'. The variety of sexual practices and preferences need no longer be seen as perversions or neurotic, but as valid ways in which a person's sexuality might be defined and expressed.

In judging the validity of such arguments, concepts used in analysing cross-cultural counselling are relevant, in particular the emic–etic and autoplastic–alloplastic axes of classification (Draguns 1981). On the emic–etic axis, the emic pole refers to the belief that psychotherapy is totally embedded in a cultural context. The opposite etic pole of the axis suggests that, for example, Western ideas are universally applicable. The auto-plastic–alloplastic axis refers to the focus of change. At the auto-plastic pole problems are changed by changing the self; at the alloplastic pole they are changed by changing the environment. The debate can therefore be characterized as a clash between etic/autoplastic and emic/alloplastic ideas (see Figure 3.1, 'Models of change'). A further difficulty in proposing the universality,

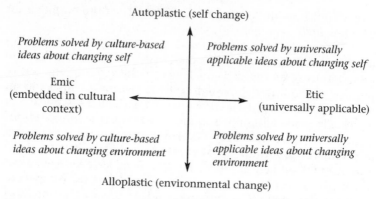

Figure 3.1 Models of change

even in Western culture, of the Oedipus complex, rooted in two heterosexual parents, lies in the fact that there are many people who do not have this experience. This includes those in one-parent families as well as those brought up in the context of gay relationships.

Lacan and the phallus

One of the main features of Lacan's interpretation of psycho-analysis is that it displaces identity and desire from biology to language. This means that he is particularly interested in the use of language, and how this relates to our experience and how it shapes our lives. In general, the concepts he develops are not easy to discuss without referring to extensive background knowledge, and this applies to his ideas about the Oedipus complex as much as to other areas of his thought. However, his ideas are too rele-vant and important to ignore, and our brief discussion will hope-fully be an encouragement to explore his ideas further. Lacan's work is a 'return to Freud' in the sense of 'an attempt to return to the spirit of the text in a modern sense, rather than an exege-sis in a historical sense' (Wilden 1968: ix). This involves recourse to the ideas that have been developed in modern linguistics as 'the science of language which allow the science of the uncon-scious to be articulated' (Lemaire 1977: xvi). The awakening of consciousness in the child is a process that takes place at the same time as the infant familiarizes himself with the use of language, which is the means by which he gradually learns about, and becomes part of, society (Lemaire 1977: 53).

Barsanti (1997) discusses how Lacan uses these language-based ideas to reinterpret Freud's Oedipal model, in a way which makes it less literally connected with ideas about anatomy and the body, and more symbolic. An example of this in everyday life is the way that the term 'pain in the neck' has developed, along-side the literal sense, a metaphorical use to refer to a difficult person. Therefore, in relation to the child's Oedipal experience, Lacan uses the term *phallus* to describe the idea that there is some-thing for ever out of the child's reach to which his mother's desire is directed (Leader and Groves 1995: 93). In this way the phallus becomes 'a symbol, representing the enjoyment that has been lost in getting through the Oedipus complex' (Leader and Groves 1995: 96). Some are uncomfortable with the place of the phallus in Lacan's thought as it seems to reinforce socially constructed gender stereotypes more than challenge them. Barsanti is un-happy about the way Lacan says that a woman desires to become the phallus, rejects her 'femininity' and pursues the phallus as her object of desire.

Sexuality for Lacan is a search for meaning and contact that provides identifications for the individual. These identifications are comforting on one level, yet on another they are a continual reminder of the loss of self that occurs when the individual becomes aware of self. This happens because, in order to have such an awareness, there has to be a split in the self, and in the course of this the self becomes an object. This leads Lacan to a pessimistic view of sexual activity, where 'individuals are not turned on by the other but by their own being turned on. For Lacan there is a fundamental alienation and narcissism within sexuality itself: the other is a mirage, a refraction of something in myself that I have lost and can never find' (Horrocks 1997: 72). Fink (1997) concludes that, for Lacan, human sexuality is funda-mentally pleasure-seeking without knowledge of higher purposes or appropriate objects. The other person is pursued because he or she has something that does something for us. This can take various forms: for example the obsessive reduces his partner to an object and the hysteric 'does not so much desire her partner as desire via her partner and wish to be the object he is lacking' (Fink 1997: 166). In this way all human desire becomes essen-tially perverse or fetishistic in nature.

One consequence of Lacan placing sexuality at the base of selfhood is that for him sexual activity is fundamentally con-cerned with identity and loss of identity. The process of sex allows for the penetration of actual physical boundaries and the disso-lution of psychological boundaries, which allows individuals to merge and re-emerge, an experience that can be pleasurable but also frightening. This may help explain why some people are unable to allow themselves to go through such an experience, where the prospect of a temporary loss of self may pose too many psychic risks. Alternatively, others may allow sex to happen, but need to defend themselves through mechanisms such as dissociation which will allow them to experience themselves as a spectator of the interaction. Although Lacan's notion of desire is one that is bound up with this existential need to define oneself, it is ultimately illusory, as 'desire always fails in its attempts to attain its object, for desire is illusory and its object is illusory. Sexual desire is saturated in fantasy, and therefore actual sex is frequently disappointing since "reality" cannot match up to fantasy' (Horrocks 1997: 74–5). Thus some people need to pursue more and more elaborate or different sexual experiences in a vain attempt to attain sexual fulfilment.

Fantasies of falling in love often involve the idea of a partner who is the perfect match in whom the very things that are lacked will be discovered in the other, and a completeness brought about. The difficulty in reality is that for most people this experience does not last, resulting in frustration and anger at the partner for failing to live up to the fantasy. However, for Lacan this is not about the need for relationship, as he has asserted that 'there is no such thing as a sexual relation' (Horrocks 1997: 74). Lacan is therefore limited in his understanding of sexual difficulties from a relationship perspective and excludes the possibility of understanding sexuality in a more positively reparative way. Also his ideas do not seem to reflect the fact that individuals can often accommodate disappointments and continue to have sexual relationships in a mutually satisfying way.

Fairbairn, Winnicott and Bion

Fairbairn (1954: 29–41) took Freud's idea of libido and changed it from an innate drive that is pleasure-seeking to a psychological entity involving the concept of a central ego seeking to relate to objects where it may find support. Libido, in this view, is essentially object-seeking, and the erotogenic zones are the means of mediating the aims of the ego. Pleasure is viewed as a 'signpost to the object' and the erotogenic zones as 'channels through which libido flows' (pp. 32–4). Ego development is conceived in terms of relationships with objects, and in particular with those internalized during the early years of life under the pressures of deprivation and frustration. In this context the individual ego is composed of a tripartite system of internal objects and parts of the self, relating dynamically to each other. The central ego and its ideal object are defended against painful and dangerous feelings by the other two parts of the system: the anti-libidinal (rejecting) part and the libidinal ego (exciting) part. Both of these parts of the ego are the result of internal struggles with split-off repressed parts of the self.

According to Fairbairn this process of internalization leads the individual to repress or deny the thoughts, affects and experiences associated with the bad object. This leaves the conscious central ego attached to the idealized core object in an attempt to form a good object relationship with which the individual can live. Examples of this ideal object would be the non-sexual, over-caring mother who is described as wonderful, and the man who is violent to his partner but is still not seen by him as bad for her. Fairbairn's exciting or libidinal object embraces sexuality as a major source of excitement. Sexual relatedness is the dynamic of excited attraction, and is a legacy of the original physical processes in early relationships. Both the child's and mother's longing for this contact is libidinal, and this partnership forms the basis for future sexual development.

Winnicott (1965) refers to this as the *psychosomatic partnership* and locates the basis for this within the primitive sensory exchanges that take place within the physical and psychological care given by the mother to the infant. He uses the term 'psychosomatic partnership' because of the intense psychological and somatic interactions that occur at this time. These provide what Winnicott (1965: 68) calls the facilitating environment, which leads to the development of internal self structures and a state of 'indwelling'. This gives the subjective sense that body and mind are integrated, rather than isolated each from the other; that the person lives in their body and yet also experiences the body as self (Winnicott 1965: 68). He hypothesized that if the baby has to develop premature ego-defences in response to an environment which fails to adapt sufficiently to the baby's needs, then this can result in mental functioning becoming a separate entity. This leads to the development of splits between different parts of the mind, and between the mind and the body:

> One of the aims of psychosomatic illness is to draw the psyche from the mind back to the original intimate association

with the soma. One has to be able to see the positive value of the somatic disturbance in its work of counteracting a 'seduction' of the psyche into the mind.

(Winnicott 1953: 254)

For the sexually functioning adult there needs to be enough internal psychological space for the individual to allow physiological responses to happen. In some ways sexual difficulties are psychologically protective, but for most individuals disruptions to their sexual functioning generate anxieties that are difficult to contain. As McDougall (1989) suggests, we may all be vulnerable to somatization when we are unable to process our fears at a mental level, where they can be modified and understood. Unexpected and unplanned external events or physiological changes through accidents or illness may well provoke unconscious processes that can affect the normal sexual response on many levels. Thus the ability to integrate sexual meaning and behaviour is part of a healthy psychic structure. On the other hand, if sensations from the body and genital awareness are repressed, vulnerability to psychosomatic disturbance can appear.

Scharff (1988) integrates the notion of sexual desire with the need-exciting libidinal ego and the longing for relationship. Developmentally, individuals move through Oedipal periods, where excitement is contained within family relationships, up to the point of puberty, when the individual increasingly focuses sexual interest externally. 'The parents respond to this sexualization with their own reactions, which reflect the quality of their internalized objects' (Scharff 1988: 50). Problems arise for individuals when their denied and repressed 'bad' experiences interfere with their ability to form healthy attachments on the necessary different levels in the present. For example, some couples are able to manage their day-to-day practical interactions, but yet on a sexual level they are unable to find mutual satisfaction. In seeing sexuality as partly a function of the internalizations that have resulted from past excitement and rejection, Scharff takes Fairbairn's ideas and applies them to sexuality and sexual problems. Sexual arousal is mediated through the ability to deal unconsciously with feelings that are provoked when the individual is sexually aroused, or wants to be sexually intimate. The degree to which individuals have to employ defence mechanisms such as projection and projective identification illustrates the extent of unconscious threat posed by these split-off experiences and feelings.

The difficulty of developing a sense of self is made problematic by the existence of powerful projections. The mother needs to be able to offer a relationship within which the infant's processes of projection can happen without the mother being damaged. The infant also needs to be able to go through a process of introjective identification with the mother in a way that is benign and growth-promoting. Introjective identification describes the means by which the functions of an external object are taken over by an internal representation which then becomes a part of the self. It is part of the developmental process by which a person becomes more autonomous. Bion describes this situation by using the concept of container-contained; the mother needs to be a strong-enough container, and the infant needs to have the experience of being contained. In containing the infant's projections the mother needs to be able to continue to tune in to the infant and respond and not withdraw.

In his work on groups, Bion identifies the tendency for the activities of a group to be based on shared unconscious assumptions which fit the unconscious needs of its members. This concept, and resultant ideas about the operation of projective identification, has been applied to families (e.g. Zinner and Shapiro 1974) and couples (Dicks 1967). Couples can be seen as operating with shared assumptions, both conscious and unconscious, particularly around attachment and separation needs. Disturbing issues surrounding these are also involved, for example anxieties about intimacy and loss. There is a tendency for the couple to create a single psychic identity by the blurring of the boundary between their distinct personalities. Within this entity the characteristics of both individuals are parcelled out by projection and introjection so that one partner may, for example, end up expressing emotion for both, or own all the intimacy needs. This means that certain perceptions of the partner are experienced as if they were part of oneself, and the partner consequently treated according to whether that aspect of self is valued or not. Projective identification is used both as a defence and a communication. As a defence, projective identification involves disowning certain parts of the self. As a communication (if it is recognized as such) it tells the partner what it feels like for the other to have a particular characteristic. In this way aspects of the self can be defended against, or managed through the interaction between two people.

This concept of projective identification originated in the work of Melanie Klein, and has been further developed to extend the psychodynamic understanding of psychological processes involved in interpersonal relationships. The dynamics of projective identification have their origins in very early experience, in the time when the child was unable to tell the difference between the self and external objects. 'In projective identification, this blurring of the self–other boundary is accompanied by the need to control the other, which comes from the early state of childhood grandiose omnipotence' (McLeod 1998: 41).

> Joseph and Masie came to therapy because Joseph developed erectile difficulties and they were unable to have a satisfactory sexual relationship. Masie complained that Joseph was angry with her, and said that this resulted in her not feeling sexual towards him. In fact he was always the one who initiated sexual contact, which allowed Masie to disown her own sexual needs and sexual feelings. Joseph, in the face of all this, was often aware of feeling confused, and sometimes was angry. Their descriptions of their interactions suggested that Masie avoided feeling angry (and sexual) by projecting her feelings unconsciously into Joseph. She accused him of being angry, and entertained doubts about whether he found her sexually attractive. In response to this Joseph would feel angry (without really being sure why) and become uncommunicative. Masie would take this as a proof of what she already believed, and Joseph would eventually enact Masie's anger by becoming angry with her. This was a relationship in which projector and recipient interacted together, unconsciously managing their problematic feelings and impulses. This process involved the blurring of boundaries between the two selves, in such a way that each individual was unaware of their own feelings and impulses.

Dicks's object-relations view of couple relationships

A psychodynamic understanding of sexual problems needs to be rooted in an understanding of how individual development leads to the potential for the couple relationship, and determines its nature. All sexual activity has a relationship dimension, even if this sometimes exists only as either phantasy objects that the person has internalized (e.g. the ideal lover or partner) or ones that he or she imagines (i.e. fantasy). Henry Dicks's *Marital Tensions*, published in 1967, is a pioneering work in the psychodynamic understanding of couple relationships, and their roots in early experiences. At that time he identified marriage as a social institution which continued to be the expression of the culture's aspiration to ensure the stability, security and dignity of relational needs between the sexes, and of children. Since then the pattern of marriage and divorce has changed considerably, but such aspirations to some kind of couple relationship are still relevant for the majority of people.

Dicks proposes that marriage (which we use to stand for the various kinds of committed couple relationship) is a system of interpersonal relations which is stable and durable to the degree that it achieves an overall positive balance of satisfactions over dissatisfactions for both partners. This does not imply either freedom from conflict nor necessarily continuous 'happiness'. The sexual relationship is a constituent part of this balance of satisfactions and dissatisfactions in the overall relationship. The long-term quality of a marriage is determined by the 'mix' and interaction of various aspects of the relationship, many of which are unconscious or barely operate at a conscious level.

Successful adaptation to a stable couple relationship requires a blend of autonomy and dependence, which are also preconditions for a good sexual relationship. A potential for autonomy presupposes an established sense of personal identity and ego strength. To develop this the child needs reciprocal relationships with people who respond in appropriate ways, not only by acceptance, but also by refusal where indicated. Acceptance confirms the child's loveableness, and refusal protects the child against feared inner impulses. The infant begins with crude experiences of 'good' (i.e. gratifying) and 'bad' (i.e. frustrating) objects (mainly parents) and advances to a gradual lessening of these apparent opposites. He or she is able to test the reality of responses, to recognize the real person of the mother, to tolerate frustration, and to contain ambivalent feelings of love and hate. From this point a feeling grows that a relationship with the outside world will be able to satisfy the infant's needs.

Dicks says that if there is a preponderance of secure, loving experiences in this testing of reality, then relational potential is created. The child internalizes the good object's feelings both as self-valuation and as a role-model and these contribute to the person's inner resources. When things work out well, the child comes to internalize a safe inner blueprint, which consists of half oneself and half love-object. Where a loving mother and father are united in cooperating to bring up the child, this also creates security, easing the child's conflicts. However, where there is parental strife, open violence and sexual frustration within the marriage, these make the child's feared fantasies into possible realities. These fantasies include his or her hate driving a wedge between the parents, stealing one parent from the other, and the parents' sex life being a violent, murderous act. In addition, in reality the parents' hate and erotic libido is likely to become directed towards one or more of the children.

If things develop in this problematic direction, the child will be left with unresolved needs in relation to parents, that otherwise might have been outgrown. These particularly take the form of ambivalent feelings of love and hate whereby 'bad' parent figures are internalized, and the whole relational potential is repressed. Where parents are experienced in this hate-arousing way, the hate is split off in the individual's internal object world in order to preserve the self. These split-off objects use psychic energy and leave less of the self available for adult relationships. Along with the hate, the need for love becomes split off, together with the child's frustrated anger. This also has to be internalized, because the child fears that the consequences of expressing it will be that the parent will be destroyed or that the infant will be rejected by the parent. These processes work together to produce a person who has conflicting forces in his or her inner world. As a result loved figures are experienced in relationships either as too punishing and castrating, or as too uncontrolled and demanding. This threatens the security of the central ego and, in response, defences are directed towards keeping the split-off ego fragments repressed.

Denying the reality of this ambivalence towards the love-object leads to projection. The partner is either seen as having the bad feelings the person cannot own, or as all good, and the person takes on all the guilt and badness. In neither instance is the partner experienced as a safe, real person. This framework can explain, through the evocation of infantile relational capacities, how difficulties in marriage can be experienced by otherwise well adjusted, successful people. Boundaries are often confused in such disturbed relationships as unconscious bonds make such couples into a unit around which joint ego boundaries are drawn, and within which they attribute to each other unconsciously shared feelings in a symbiotic or collusive process. This enables us to understand why some couples stay together despite every appearance of suffering and mutual destructiveness in the relationship. For example, a person may persecute a spouse for traits that were originally attractive, the spouse having been unconsciously perceived as symbolizing what had been repressed (and therefore lost) in the person's self. The partner is then treated as if he or she were indeed this aspect of the self – i.e. first cherished and then persecuted.

The main defence within marriage identified by Dicks is idealization – the idea that the partner must be perfect, make good all defects, and offer complete gratification. Idealization involves the repression of the hate side of ambivalence. Many tensions and misunderstandings result from disappointment when the partner fails to play a role corresponding to the person's fantasy world. If idealization breaks down, repressed hate towards parent figures is activated. In such marriages there is an inability to tolerate such aspects as anger or boredom within the relationship. There is also a denial of the freedom of the other to deviate from the ideal image.

Couples who continue to live in states of severe conflict and mutual frustration appear not to have given up the struggle to come to terms with and work through their inner object world. In a happy marriage the inner contents of the dyad consist of predominantly good objects. In problem marriages the same sense of belonging provides the opportunity to share and inflict on partners highly ambivalent infantile object relations that need such expression. One form of this is the schizoid position as described by Klein and Fairbairn, where loving and being loved have become identified with destroying and being destroyed. Consequently the only safe thing is to act towards the libidinal object in a way that will drive it away to avoid damaging it or to avoid being damaged, or even devoured, by it. This leads to hateful communication, and at the same time a craving for infantile dependence and support.

The couple relationship as container

In thinking about the couple relationship as a psychological container it is important to keep in mind each partner's internal worlds and the dynamics of the couple relationship (Colman 1993a: 72). Jung was the first to describe marriage as an emotional container (Jung 1925). This containment can be thought of in three ways. The marriage itself is a container in terms of the commitment made, while each partner both contains the other and is contained by them (Lyons and Mattinson 1993: 107). Colman (1993b: 129) says that:

> Jung's idea of the psyche as a self-regulating system based on the balance of opposites is similar to the family systems notion of homeostasis, the way in which a family strives to achieve a workable balance between its opposing forces. This is another way of stating the developmental potential of marriage, since, if it is to be successful, it requires the capacity to sustain the tensions arising from a whole host of oppositions – e.g. my needs vs. your needs, separateness vs. togetherness, autonomy vs. dependence, love vs. hate, exploration vs. safety, similarity vs. difference, and, indeed, defence vs. development – the list is potentially endless.

The role of defences in couple relationships

Pincus also emphasizes the importance of idealization as a defence in marriage, but sees projection as an equally important defence in couple relationships. In extreme situations so much can be projected that the one personality may become impoverished while the other is invaded. Where this happens in a couple relationship anxiety is caused by having to maintain this situation:

> The relation with the person who is thus invaded partly becomes a relationship with the self, and the partner ceases to exist as an individual in his own right. Where the pattern of defences is excessively fragile or too rigid, each partner may cling to a false image of himself and the other, and reality-testing, which makes for growth and development, becomes impossible. The more this happens, the greater will be the pressure to maintain a situation in which the rejected parts are completely split off from the rest of the personality.

> (Pincus 1976: 35–6)

Daniell (1985) says that although partners may consciously choose each other for their 'good' qualities, often unconsciously they choose someone with a shared level of immaturity. Where this shared immaturity is not too great, it may prove helpful, if partners can provide each other with the time, space and trust to work through their shared area of disturbance. Where there are greater difficulties, there often exists collusion between partners to maintain mutual or complementary defences based on a shared fantasy about the catastrophe that will result if feared or unacceptable impulses in the self and in the partner are allowed to emerge. The way these defences are set up means that in therapy with couples it frequently becomes apparent that what was at first attractive, and is later complained of, is a projection of unwanted and repudiated parts of the self. Couple relationships based on these kinds of mutually defensive systems that work initially may become disturbed when a major change in lifestyle takes place.

> Liz had recently been made redundant from her job as a librarian, and had become quite depressed about her future employment prospects. She had been living in a lesbian relationship with Meera for the past three years. They described their relationship as rocky, with sex being almost non-existent. They both spent the first session saying that the other was the problem. Meera complained that Liz was untidy and selfish, being preoccupied only with how she felt. Liz complained that Meera was fussy, overbearing and insecure. When they were asked individually to describe what attracted each of them to the other, it emerged that Meera found Liz independent and strong, and not frightened to speak her mind and express her feelings; whereas Liz thought that Meera was attentive and careful, and she liked the fact that she appeared quite vulnerable. The very qualities that they had found attractive in each other were now causing problems. Liz had become financially dependent on Meera, which had disrupted their original mutual defence system, whereby they both unconsciously projected unwanted aspects of themselves onto the other. Meera had projected her aggressive independent aspect onto Liz, and Liz had projected her needy vulnerable self onto Meera.

Sexual function is in varying degrees influenced by the dynamics of the interaction with others on both a conscious and unconscious level. For example, some will recount how their sexual difficulty occurs in one relationship and not in others. This might be understood in a number of ways, including the effect of unconscious projections between partners. At each developmental stage the parents' awareness of the child's emotional, physical and educational needs has a significant influence on the course of sexual development and adjustment. The ability, for example, of the adolescent to masturbate with pleasure and without guilt has the effect of strengthening the original psychosomatic relationship while allowing the potential for later adult sexual experiences and relationships.

Conclusion

We have outlined the relevant concepts which might underpin a psychodynamic theory of sexual problems, starting from Freud and working through to the modern object-relations writers. This emphasis, on the dynamic and symbolic nature of sexual interaction, involves not only a physical interaction, but also an emotional link between two people each with their own internal set of object relationships constituting their emotional world. In the next chapter we can further explore the ways in which these concepts relate to an understanding of sexuality and sexual difficulties.

Chapter 4

A *psychodynamic approach to sexuality and sexual problems*

In this chapter we shall lay a foundation of theoretical concepts upon which we can build a psychodynamic process of assessing and treating sexual problems. There are a number of ways in which counsellors may wish to use psychodynamic ideas in relation to sexuality and sexual problems. Some use psychodynamic understandings and insights, but do not necessarily employ these directly in therapy. Other counsellors use such understandings as part of an integrative approach, incorporating psychodynamic ideas and interventions with those deriving from other theoretical perspectives. These perspectives can be broader than just other counselling theories and, for example, can include physical treatments used to treat sexual symptoms. Counsellors who work entirely in a psychodynamic way may wish to increase their understanding and effectiveness in working with the sexual problems presented by their clients.

Some comments on integrating approaches

Many counsellors working with sexual problems combine components of different approaches in their work, including aspects of psychodynamic ways of working. Many clients present with specific sexual problems for which behavioural and cognitive techniques can bring about effective change in a short period, but others do not respond well to such programmes. Psychodynamic understanding of the way phantasies and defences operate between couples and form part of the transference with the therapist can be a valuable key in unlocking such situations. Therefore a purely psychodynamic approach, integrating a psychodynamic approach with physical treatments, or using psychodynamic ideas with other theories, may be the only way to enable some individuals and couples to make lasting changes in their sexual relating.

Some counsellors develop their approach mainly on a pragmatic basis, incorporating 'what works', but there is a strong argument that a firm theoretical basis should underlie such an enterprise. Without this a counsellor can drift into deploying concurrent techniques without regard for their theoretical origins or conceptual implications. In developing an integrated approach there is a danger of assuming that all kinds of intervention can be effectively used together. It is important to recognize that they can potentially cancel each other out as well as complement each other. For instance, the use of directive techniques makes person-centred non-directiveness impossible. Additionally the effect of an intervention changes according to the context in which it appears. Therefore a task set within a behavioural understanding of the situation may be experienced as persecutory if it is suddenly introduced into a session that has up to then operated within a psychodynamic framework.

A number of ways of integrating theories and practice have been used with sexual and couple relationship problems. There are approaches that use clinical interventions predominantly from one approach, but draw on more than one theory. An example of this is Segraves (1982), who uses a predominantly cognitive approach which also draws on psychodynamic theory. Some of the complications of integration are avoided by sequential approaches, starting by using one approach, and following it by a more complex approach if the first does not work. Crowe and Ridley (1990) propose the use of behavioural followed by systemic interventions, and Daines (1992: 72–3) looks at the possibility of developing a sequential behavioural-psychodynamic approach. A more complex possibility is multi-theory followed by multi-practice, an example of which is Skynner's (e.g. 1976) use of psychodynamic and systemic theory leading to mainly systemic, but also group analytic interventions. Some practitioners use a single theory followed by clinical interventions drawing on more than one set of clinical interventions. For example, the Institute of Psychosexual Medicine uses predominantly psychoanalytic ideas in its theory, but is behavioural as well as analytic in its clinical practices. Finally there are fully integrated approaches, which involve the theoretical concepts and practices of more than one theory, used together. The Relate approach is an example of this (e.g. Sandford and Beardsley 1986). There are numerous possibilities, most of which have complex issues attached to their development and usage. Those who wish to use psychodynamic ideas as part of an integrated approach need to consider the psychodynamic implications of the other integrated components.

> A client complained to his therapist of having a small and painful penis, and a medical colleague was asked, with the man's permission, to give a physical examination of the problem. This examination revealed that the man had an average size penis, but that his foreskin was retracted and inflamed, and needed antibiotic medication. During the subsequent psychotherapy sessions it was necessary to return again and again to this examination. It showed more clearly to the client that his difficulties, and the way that his phantasies about his inadequate penis operated, kept him from being able to form relationships. The physical examination provoked many strong feelings within this man, and it became obvious that he used projection of both negative and positive parts of himself. Working within the transference enabled him to understand this, and how his relationship with his parents was related to his current feelings, all of which had been stimulated by the therapist and the doctor.

Trying to understand integrated approaches as they are used in practice is further complicated by the fact that therapists may or may not act in the way that they theoretically describe (Maguire 1973). Additionally clients' perceptions may be very different from those intended by the therapists, and their subjective experience very different from that described in counselling or psychotherapy theory. Ultimately there is a need for combining approaches, not as a process of dilution or contamination, but rather as a creative act, leading to work with clients that can be justified both theoretically and practically.

Working within a time-limited framework

Psychodynamic work with sexual difficulties can be practised with an open-ended contract or as a form of time-limited psychotherapy. Sandor Ferenczi and Otto Rank were among the earliest to challenge traditional psychoanalytic techniques, proposing that therapy can be time limited and that the therapist can be more active during the process. These ideas form the background to the development of the theory and practice of time-limited psychodynamic therapy, its application to specific kinds of psychological difficulties, and its relevance to certain settings. Some of the pressure for this development has arisen from social and economic factors, especially in the public sector where therapists of all orientations have needed to examine the most cost-effective way of using limited resources. Sex therapy work within the NHS has been part of this.

While time-limited work is not suitable for all situations, a wide range of sexual problems can be worked with in this way, as such difficulties provide a suitable focus for the work. Where a number of different kinds of difficulties are presented, clients should be encouraged to decide with the therapist if the sexual problem is the most suitable focus. For example, with clients who have been sexually abused, it is necessary to assess with the client how far their current sexual problem can be the central issue in the therapeutic work, or how much it needs to be the sexual abuse.

In this way time-limited work has a more active style, involving more specific negotiation with clients about the aims and expectations of psychotherapy in relation to their difficulties. Clearly clients who cannot participate in such a dialogue are not suitable for time-limited work. A more active style by the therapist enables limited interpretations to be offered early on in the process (Malan 1976; Gustafson 1986). This contrasts with traditional psychoanalytic work where themes and associations are allowed to develop at their own pace and the analyst offers a 'blank screen' upon which the projected transferences can be analysed. In time-limited work the therapist needs to work actively with the transference as early as possible. The limited time frame itself helps this process as it can generate both positive and negative transferential reactions. Examples of these reactions include the feeling that there is not enough time, or a sense of relief that there is not the opportunity to become very dependent on the therapist: such responses contribute to the interpretations that can be made. Further, the sexual nature of the material can generate degrees of excitement or anxiety in the client that need to be commented upon immediately. Fantasies abound in clients about what might happen to them when they ask for help with sexual problems, which relate to interactions between their internal fantasies and common misconceptions about sex therapy. It is helpful to the progress of the work if these anxieties and fantasies are explored early in time-imited work, otherwise they may impede the client's progress.

> An elderly man called Roy presented with worries about premature ejaculation. He was sexually inexperienced, and when aroused his penis allowed a small amount of pre-ejaculate to escape, which Roy believed to be a full ejaculation. This apparent loss of control was interfering with his sexual relationship with a close woman friend. During the second session Roy became acutely embarrassed and, after some difficulty, explained that he was not sure why he was coming for help, an attitude in sharp contrast to that at the previous session. It was suggested to him that he appeared to be under some pressure to leave before he had given himself the chance to look at his difficulties, and that it was not clear what this was about.
>
> It transpired that he had interpreted questions about masturbation asked at the assessment interview as an instruction to masturbate. This literal interpretation arose from a combination of his conscious and unexplored ideas about sex therapy, and an unconscious inner world of controlling and anxiety-provoking objects. His reactions gave the therapist the opportunity to explore his fantasies about sex therapy, and the need to set clear boundaries about expectations. This process contained Roy's fears and projections and enabled him safely to explore his sexual difficulties without undue anxiety or feeling out of control.

Time-limited psychodynamic work is useful with clients who are motivated and able to have insights into their sexual difficulties which will allow them to make changes. One of the benefits of working in this way is that it encourages clients to integrate and understand the impact of a number of factors on their sexual problem, both conscious and unconscious. The main exceptions to this are where such problems form part of a complex set of psychological difficulties, as in the following example, or where clients wish to work in a less focused way and are able to benefit from this.

> Trudie presented at the assessment interview complaining that she could not have an orgasm. During this interview

she was asked about her relationship, and the therapist noted that she did not have anyone she would describe as a friend. She maintained that her job as a consultant orthodontist restricted her in making friends. She also had a complete absence of family relationships, and little sense of herself other than in her work role. Not surprisingly she had never been able to form a sexual relationship over any extended period of time. By the third session she was becoming quite withdrawn and monosyllabic, clearly finding relating to the therapist difficult. At this point it emerged that she needed long-term work to help her address her difficulties that were central to her sense of self. The sexual problem was a manifestation of quite severe psychological problems that were revealed as she struggled in her relationship with the therapist.

There are also clients who do not want to work in a time-limited way, who perhaps find it difficult to focus, who want time to explore things, or who feel too pressurized by the time limit to be able to work on their problems. Therefore an important part of the assessment process is to explore this possibility and reach an agreement about the suitability of the time frame. Writers on time-limited psychodynamic work have different ideas about what actual time scale needs to be used and discuss different styles of brief psychodynamic work that have been evolved (see Malan 1976, 1979; Gustafson 1986). There is, however, a general agreement that time-limited work is focused on three discrete stages: the beginning, the active phase and the termination (Rosen 1987). Generally the set number of sessions is up to 25, with the agreement about number made clear at the start.

Psychodynamic processes underlying sexual activity

Before going on to consider the psychodynamic processes that produce sexual difficulties, first of all we need to establish some of the main psychodynamic processes underlying sexual activity. Many writers are more interested in the mechanisms producing sexual dysfunctions than in exploring those that are essential for a satisfactory sex life. However, returning to the idea of the psychosomatic partnership discussed in Chapter 3, Scharff shows how this links in with adult sexual relationships:

If we approach the sexual relationship as a psychosomatic partnership, we can map out the way these specific interactions between bodies – between genitalia, breasts, mouths, hands – express and speak to profound emotional relationships. The adult sexual relationship is in part a replay of early relationships, which lends it a poignancy that few other relationships approach. In this setting, sexuality taps into the need-exciting object constellation, whilst sexual rejection and frustration resonate with rejecting object systems. The internal object relations that represent these tend to recreate these experiences in interaction with the external object, and a sexually heightened body experience of them magnifies their unconscious role for each of the participants. It is in these ways that adult sexuality is the inheritor of the earlier mother–infant psychosomatic partnership.

(Scharff 1982: 121)

He draws extensively on the thinking of Fairbairn and of Klein in providing a framework for understanding adult sexual relationships. He says that:

a physical sexual relationship draws . . . on the internalised aspects of past relationships, giving them new life and providing an opportunity for reworking these old relationships in the context of the present ones. Adult sexual ties thereby unite the images and memories of the past family with the experience of the current family, revising and preserving the past in a new context.

(p. 1)

In adult life, childhood needs are split off, so that gratification happens in vicarious and symbolic ways. However, sexuality can renew the 'old bond between the physical and symbolic levels of gratification, reviving the childhood developmental conflicts of the individual and transiently permitting more direct gratification' (p. 4).

In the meeting of the couple's sexual needs a bridge is formed, not just between their object worlds but also between the soma and psyche within each of them. This bridge provides each person with new opportunities to rework old issues. This is the medium through which sexual problems can be generated. The erotic zone operates as a kind of projection screen, making it the physical locus of conflicts with internalized objects and current primary figures. Sex therefore becomes a sign which symbolizes an internal sense of well-being, through the link with good internal objects (or conversely a lack of sense of well-being through a link with bad internal objects). Symbolically it comes to stand for the struggle to hold on to the memory of the giving loving parent. It helps overcome the image of the withholding parent by synthesizing and repairing these two images.

> Karen and Phillip had been married for three years and came to therapy because of Karen's loss of libido, which was caused by her having dyspareunia. She had always found sex painful and they had both become distressed about this. Increasingly they both felt something very important was missing from their relationship, and they had both become pessimistic about being able to change the situation. They had both known each other for many years before marrying, as their families were friendly with each other. Both families continued to be supportive to them. Phillip was the youngest of two in what he described as a normal working-class family. He described his father as very much a family man and his mother as having a tendency to worry too much. Karen characterized her parents as 'lovely people who would do anything for anyone'. Both sets of parents had high expectations of them, and were looking forward to their producing grandchildren.
>
> Karen and Phillip attended for 25 sessions in total. At around session 16 Karen talked about how bad she felt as a person, not only for letting Phillip down but also her parents. She expressed her upset about not even being able to make therapy work and how she could understand if both Phillip and the therapist could not cope with her any more. In response to this Phillip became anxious and tried to reassure Karen that everything would work out. This resulted in Karen becoming angry with him and accusing him of being too reasonable. Phillip withdrew in response to this attack, not being sure what to say. Karen then began to express more clearly her fears that they would not be able to sort out their problems. It was as if the sexual difficulty represented the crack in a perfect relationship, an image which they were struggling to maintain both between themselves and to the outside world. Both Karen's and Phillip's internal worlds were populated by images of perfect, flawless relationships. Unconsciously

they had both sought out a partner that would enable them to re-create this sense of perfection.

Her frustration with Phillip's reasonableness was the start of consciously working through their less-than-perfect feelings for each other. They also acknowledged the pressure that they felt to live up to their parents' expectations, which fitted their internalized picture of what relationships should be like. Their work on emotionally separating from this became clear when they announced to their parents that they would not be having children in the immediate future. Their ability to contain difference and disagreement improved, as did their frustration that their marriage and their sexual relationship were not flawless.

The psychodynamic nature of sexuality and the ability to engage in relationships is looked at further by Scharff, who goes on to develop a framework where 'the maturity of sexual relatedness is an achievement resting on the balance between the individual, his internal objects, and his external relationships' (Scharff 1982: 214). At the most basic level sexual interest stems from an interest in one's own body. This has its roots in early attachment experiences and therefore comes to represent a wish to establish intimacy in the face of loss or separation. Sexual interest also stems from Oedipal relationships, in particular the resolution of the tensions caused by the internalization of both the exciting mother and the rejecting mother (see Scharff 1982: 71). A successful resolution forms the basis for cooperation and mutual sexual satisfaction between the couple, and the later sublimated investment in children, in work and emotional growth together.

During sexual activity individuals move through a series of conscious and unconscious thoughts, feelings and actions that are integral to their ability to be able to function sexually. Sex is an opportunity for the individual to differentiate and process somatic and verbal expressions. This ability to process conscious and unconscious aspects of these experiences and convert them to 'language' is influenced by the adult's earliest interactions as a baby with its caregiver. Edgecumbe (1985) has pointed out that the first differentiation that an infant makes (with the help of the mother) is between the experience of something happening and his own response to it. Further development involves the differentiation of experience into somatic and psychic, and there are further divisions into thoughts, feelings and actions, and so on.

Overall the two main forms of expression remain the verbal and the bodily. Their significance depends on the value that they have acquired within the mother–child relationship, and their representation in the child's inner world:

> Body language comprises somatic symptoms and physical actions; verbal language includes the various levels of thought and fantasy. Emotions, and perhaps some levels of non-verbal fantasy, may be viewed as bridging the gap between the bodily and the mental in normal development.
>
> (Schachter 1997: 213)

Communicating in this way forms part of both the language and actuality of the sexual interaction. Sexual behaviours contain a myriad of expressions and responses, which the other partner 'reads' and to which they respond, sometimes provoking defensive reactions that can help or hinder the sexual experience.

Sexual activity of all kinds inevitably includes the expression of defences and defensive processes. Provided the sexual relationship is not required to contain too much (or too many) of these, there is no automatic reason why they should be disruptive or cause sexual dysfunctions. Therefore a certain level of containment, and possibly working through, of defences may best be considered part of normal sexual relating. At its most positive, sexual activity can be seen as *reparative*, reducing guilt by the action of making good the harm done to an object seen as both good and bad. 'Successful sexual performance constitutes both an actual and a symbolic reparation, a reinfusion of loving from the body to the multiple sources of physical and emotional needs' (Scharff and Scharff 1991: 12–13). Others, such as Klein, see sexual activity as the normal process by which the individual resolves inherent ambivalence towards objects. As such sex can be a way of dealing with ambivalence in couple relationships.

The idea of *regression* is inherent in Scharff's idea of sex reviving the 'old bond between the physical and symbolic levels of gratification' (1982: 4). Playfulness in sexual relationships has its basis in regression. *Identification* is relevant in all its three meanings: extending one's identity *into* someone else, borrowing identity *from* someone else, and fusing or confusing identity *with* someone else. These processes in sex with a partner may provide relief from preoccupations, problems and distress. Similar benefits may operate from processes of projection (whereby aspects of the self are imagined to be in the other person) and projective identification (where the self is imagined to be inside someone else).

Psychodynamic processes underlying sexual difficulties

Where the defences that underlie sexual relationships become too prominent they can be the cause of a sexual problem. Daniell says that individuals

> adopt various defensive mechanisms in order to control what they feel to be unacceptable impulses or to avoid psychic pain. In marriages there is frequently a collusion – an unconscious agreement – between the partners to maintain mutual or complementary defences. This arises from a shared fantasy about the catastrophe which will result if the feared or unacceptable impulses in the self and in the partner emerge. In marital disturbance these distorted perceptions, arising from each partner's past experiences, can frequently be rigidly held and not mediated in the light of present circumstances and experience.
>
> (Daniell 1985: 175)

The longings that underlie these defences are elaborated by Cleavely:

> At the very core of every defensive system and of every emotional conflict lies the longing for a close intimate relationship with a significant other, and of being a self-sufficient 'I' – independent, autonomous, certain of being able to survive alone. The longing, however, is associated with anxiety. For the longing for closeness arouses the fear of being 'swallowed up', taken over, dominated by the other, leading to a loss of self. The longing for autonomy gives rise to fears of being abandoned, of being destructive, of survival threatened, and the loss of the other. In the face of such conflict, ambivalence is born, and ways have to be found of managing loving and hating the same person.
>
> (Cleavely 1993: 59)

The case history below illustrates Schachter's idea that once a disease is triggered or activated, then the individual is changed both physiologically and psychologically. 'This important point may get forgotten in some purely psychoanalytic explanations of psychosomatic illness, when the unconscious fantasies which become attached secondarily to the somatic symptoms are seen as the aetiological factors' (Schachter 1997: 215).

> Bernard, aged 56, complained that he could no longer achieve a good erection and was worried about what might be wrong. He described his relationship with his wife Kaye as satisfactory, and there appeared to be no particular problems in other areas of his life. After a series of physical tests that revealed no abnormalities he attended for further assessment with his partner. She was for the most part quiet during the interview and, when encouraged to describe her perception of the situation, said that she had not seen any noticeable changes in her partner's erections. As the conversation progressed the man became very uncomfortable and Kaye again became quiet and looked puzzled. The therapist suggested that there might be some difficulty for them in discussing their problems when they had such differing perceptions. At this point Bernard became angry and accused the therapist of agreeing with his partner that he must be inadequate sexually.
>
> Kaye denied thinking in this way, and seemed perplexed at her husband's outburst. The husband described how difficult it was for him to be sure whether his wife was enjoying their lovemaking as she was always so quiet. In fact he could list a catalogue of events during lovemaking over the years that indicated to him that she believed he was sexually inadequate. Now he was not able to achieve an erection his anxieties seemed out of control. Kaye found discussing sexual matters difficult and her lack of response seemed to illustrate her difficulties, and she said she had relied heavily on Bernard knowing what was best for them sexually. In fact she often felt inadequate about not being able to say or to show him what she liked sexually. Consequently she stayed quiet to avoid thinking about such matters, and in this way thought that she would avoid upsetting Bernard. This status quo had recently come to a head for both of them when he started having erection difficulties and the sexual relationship needed to be talked about.
>
> They both carried a great deal of anxiety about sex and projected this onto each other. They had formed a

relationship which was based on their emotional immaturity. Kaye's idealization of Bernard kept her unable to think and speak for herself, especially in matters sexual. Bernard's unspoken fears about his sexual ability revealed his anxieties about his relationship and his fears about separation. Unconsciously they had both created a relationship that contained these projections, but Bernard's erection difficulties had started to undermine this arrangement. The sexual symptoms needed to be processed and understood, and the couple relationship supported, to enable them to adapt to the changes that were inextricably linked to growing older.

Traditionally, within classical psychoanalysis, the approach to sexual difficulties would be to work back to the source of these conflicts and anxieties by exposing and working through repressed material, particularly Oedipal themes, in order to benefit the current relationship (Bowen 1972; Framo 1976). This enables the individual to deal with their split-off needs and feelings, and to resolve their sublimated developmental difficulties to enable them to move on to the next stage. However, various authors (Framo 1965; Dicks 1967; Meissner 1978), in reviewing the work of various psychoanalysts, have been critical of this approach. For example, Ransom states that 'one gets the idea that people do not really relate to one another, but to ghosts, and that they are not in love with one another, but with projected aspects of their unfilled love for their parents' (Ransom 1980: 246). This criticism, that relationships get reduced to the ghosts of the past, is probably part of the reason why psychoanalytically orientated therapies have lost ground with therapies that deal with the present difficulties.

Current sexual difficulties may to varying degrees contain or illustrate earlier unresolved childhood conflicts. Both external and internal changes in people, and their relationships, interact psychodynamically to affect sexual functioning. However, working with the psychodynamic processes that are apparent in the *current* situation provides an opportunity for the present relationship to contain, understand and integrate unexpressed feelings and fears. It is possible to work with the presenting sexual symptoms, whatever their origin, in terms of highly symbolic and powerful reactions. In this way the original childhood causal conditions may be directly influenced by working with the present sexual problem, as reparation is made possible by working through the psychodynamics of the current situation (see Wile 1993: 89).

A couple in their late forties were referred by their GP to the local sex and relationship clinic. The referral was because of the female partner's 'excessive' sexual demands. At the assessment the couple described their present situation as very happy except for their rows about sex. They both enjoyed sex and felt that there were no problems with their sexual relationship itself, except that they disagreed about how often it should happen. Robert was quite happy with once or twice a week, while his partner Irene felt that ideally she would like to have sex three times a day but that once a day would be manageable. Irene was feeling very distressed that Robert did not feel the same as herself, whereas Robert thought that Irene was being totally unreasonable. This situation had existed for some time, but in the last year they both felt that they had argued more about the situation.

Robert explained that he had a busy job and tried to make as much time for their relationship as possible, but felt that this was never enough for Irene. She also had a busy life, working as a dinner lady as well as looking after her daughter's children. They came from large families, and were both the eldest child. Robert and Irene each summarized their childhood as being fairly ordinary. Irene did not attend school much as she was looking after her siblings while her mother worked. Robert left school early to work in a tool factory. He described himself as the 'apple of his mother's eye', at which point Irene snorted and claimed that was still the case. Irene on the other hand felt that she had needed to be the mother in her family, as both her parents worked. She had left home at 17 to marry Robert, whom she had met at church and then fallen in love with. They had two adult children who were now married with their own families.

During the discussion Irene described her job as fairly boring and referred to the fact that Robert had recently been promoted, and was now working later and later. She worried about this, and feared that Robert would find someone younger and more interesting. Robert's response to this was to ignore Irene's enquiries and comments about work, and to tell her as little as possible to avoid any rows. This had caused bad feeling between them, and Irene had begun to feel quite paranoid about where Robert was when he was late home. Irene took Robert's refusal to have sex as an indication that something was wrong. In fact their disagreement over sex had escalated during this time, and Irene had become angry with Robert when he refused to make love. This in turn had worried her, and she had sought mediation from her GP to control her temper.

The therapy focused on helping the couple understand and contain the different thoughts, feelings and fantasies about their relationship, in particular their sexual relationship, revealing the extent to which for both of them it symbolized their security needs for each other. It was suggested to Irene that perhaps her insecurities stemmed from being the eldest in a large family where she was expected to put others first; whereas Robert had the experience of being the centre of attention from both his parents. As successive children were born to her mother, she was put in an untenable position. Her inner demands and feelings had to be repressed or split off from an early age in order for her to be the mature helpmate that her parents relied on. In this indirect way she did obtain some acknowledgement and attention, but at the cost of not feeling entitled to her own feelings and needs. Within the relationship with Robert these had re-emerged in a distorted form via the sexual relationship, where she was continually acting out her profound fear of loss of her internal love-object. Robert for his part had married someone who would continue to idealize him as his mother did, so that he would never have to face his fears of loss; in a paradoxical way Irene's sexual demands achieved this for him.

In this case the traditional route of trying to help Irene resolve her childhood conflicts to obtain a beneficial effect upon the current relationship was not followed. By working on the current relationship, to facilitate containment and integration of her previously split-off envious feelings, the pressure on their sex life was eased. They both needed to understand how their behaviour and reactions were supporting the regeneration of Irene's earlier insecurities, at the same time reinforcing a familiar protective position for Robert. Irene had the familiar experience of not feeling entitled to have her needs met. It was understandable that she would feel envious of Robert but, instead of viewing this as pathological, they were encouraged to consider how best to support Irene to make some positive choices about her life. Once Irene had resolved her envious feelings in the context of the difficulties she was experiencing, it was then possible that she could do this with others, reworking earlier conflicts through the experience of having her needs directly met in the present relationship.

Scharff and Scharff (1991: 55) say that in sexual relationships the body becomes a medium for projection so that conflicts 'are projected in condensed form on the body screen of the genitalia'. An example of the way in which Oedipal issues play a part in the development of a sexual difficulty is shown by Hiller (1993: 17), who draws on the ideas of Ogden:

> I suggest that the collapse of the physiological reflex of the erectile response represents an internal collapse into a dyadic relationship with the mother of the pre-genital early holding environment: the inability to sustain an erection to intra-vaginal containment represents the lack of containment in the transitional oedipal relationship for the boy's secure attribution of phallic meaning to his penis: the fear of sexual failure represents the failure of the parental environment to facilitate adequate male sexual identification, either with the mother's unconscious oedipal father or with the actual father at a later stage of development.

A schema

It is now possible to set out a schema for the psychodynamic processes underlying commonly presenting sexual difficulties. This is summarized in Table 4.1 and expanded in the subsections that follow.

Problems that are primarily effects of early development

Gender identity problems

Where people come for help with issues surrounding gender identity, a psychodynamic understanding assumes that the roots of this might be found fairly early in the developmental process. Some clients may only need an opportunity for clarification of their thoughts and feelings, but the implication of locating the origin of their difficulties in early life is that for many

Table 4.1 Psychodynamic processes underlying sexual difficulties

---

Problems which are primarily effects of early development
- Gender identity problems
- Difficulties surrounding object choice
    sexual orientation
    sexual interests and preferences
- Schizoid fears of engulfment and loneliness
- Conflicts between the need to merge and the need to differentiate
- Expressions of sadism or masochism
- Emotional immaturity expressed through partner choice

Problems associated with defence mechanisms (after Bateman and Holmes 1995)
- Primitive/immature
    narcissism
    splitting
    idealization
    introjection
    projection
    projective identification
- Neurotic
    denial
    dissociation
    identification
    intellectualization
    rationalization
    reaction formation
    regression
    repression
    reversal
    somatization
- Mature
    humour
    sublimation

---

people, medium- or long-term counselling or therapy may be needed.

Difficulties surrounding object choice

Exploration or clarification of sexual preferences may be possible in a small number of sessions, but this will not be sufficient to meet the needs of many of the clients who are struggling over issues surrounding the object of their erotic desire. Some may wish to look at issues of *sexual orientation*. Others may need to look at other aspects of *sexual interests and preferences,* such as fetishism.

Schizoid fears of engulfment and loneliness

The conflicting schizoid fears of engulfment and loneliness have a profound effect on close relationships. Guntrip describes as 'the schizoid compromise' when the person 'hovers between two opposite fears, the fear of isolation in independence with loss of his ego in a vacuum of experience, and the fear of bondage to, of imprisonment or absorption in the personality of whomsoever he rushes to for protection' (Guntrip 1968: 291). Where there is a protracted schizoid problem, long-term counselling or psychotherapy is likely to be needed. Such difficulties are likely to include sexual problems. For example Guntrip (p. 44) describes a woman who saw sexual relations as only an experience and could not connect with any idea of love, or with herself as a person. In another instance he relates how guilt, which can be part of the defences of a schizoid person, led a male client to feel he ought not to experience gratification or comfort from his sexual relationship with his wife, but rather to experience sex as mechanical (p. 159). Another man 'could not respond with any sexual feeling to a woman of whom he had grown truly fond' (p. 276). McDougall talks about those who use sexuality as a drug so that sexuality 'has a compulsive and drug-like quality in that the partner plays little role in the subject's inner world, being more an object of need than an object of desire' (McDougall 1989: 99). For such people sex may be mainly a sleeping pill. 'Such partnerships may be relatively long-lasting, as long as the "sleeping pill" does not object to his/her role' (p. 99). The partner may in this way represent an object of consummation rather than another human being.

Conflicts between the need to merge and the need to differentiate

Most people have schizoid elements that are far less pronounced, but become expressed in conflicts between the need to be close and the need to be separate. It is not uncommon for one partner to want more *emotional* closeness than the other, who wishes for more *sexual* closeness than his or her partner. Such couples commonly present with difficulties about sexual interest. This can happen at the point where they make a more definite commitment within a relationship where the sexual relationship has been satisfactory. Scharff and Scharff describe the possible mechanism by which this happens:

> When it is the case that one or both partners have rather fragile excited object sets, the rejecting object and ego can now swamp the excitement and sexualization of bonding. It is for this reason that we frequently see a marked decrease of interest in sex at the moment of marriage or of commitment. A man or woman who is threatened, consciously or unconsciously, by sex because it is associated with frightening object relatedness may well muster a sexual response with pleasure under the conditions of courtship and bond making, only to have those feelings disappear once the bond seems secured.
>
> (Scharff and Scharff 1991: 26)

It is as if the individual needs to withdraw into non-sexual relating in order to protect themselves against being overwhelmed. The sexual intimacy in this way is unconsciously experienced as a threat to the self. It is also true that a lack of intimacy can make the individual feel like they do not exist. The delicate balance between these two threats is negotiated unconsciously, and not surprisingly it is often acted out through the way that couples organize their lives together. For example, couples often complain that their work and family commitments do not enable them to have sufficient time together. Such factors are used to regulate the level of closeness and distance in the relationship.

> Terry and Joanne, a young couple in their twenties recently married, presented with non-consummation of their marriage. They had during their courtship lived two hundred miles apart and had seen each other at alternate weekends, when they were able to have sex successfully. Since they had been married and living together Joanne had developed secondary vaginismus, which had prevented them from being able to have penetrative sex. She described how the relationship was wonderful prior to their marriage, but since she had moved in with her partner everything had changed. They were also feeling cheated that the very thing they had both worked so hard towards achieving was not turning out as they imagined. After four appointments, during which very little progress was achieved, it was

agreed that Joanne and Terry would each see one of the co-therapy therapists separately for one session.

During her session Joanne admitted to not feeling very sexual towards Terry since they had moved in together, and she felt desperate that her feelings had changed. In fact she came to realize that even talking about her feelings with Terry in the room made her feel panicky, suffocated and stifled. Terry for his part felt desperate and he was finding it difficult to stay calm about the situation. Once their individual stories were heard it became clear that they both had difficulties in setting personal boundaries and that this was related to the fact that they both came from families where they felt heavily pressurized to meet their parents' emotional needs. While they lived separately they were able to cope with the emotional pressure from each other and their families. Since moving in together Joanne felt that she was in danger of losing her identity, especially as Terry and their respective parents were expectantly waiting for grandchildren. Joanne realized that she did not feel ready for this, but feared Terry's reaction to her views.

Expressions of sadism or masochism

It is stating the obvious to say that sex is a common means by which sadistic and masochistic impulses can be acted out. In a minor way, between consenting adults, these may be exciting and emotionally releasing ways of creating and sustaining interest in a sexual relationship. However, to the extent that they become destructive or instruments of hate, they are likely to be experienced as distasteful, unhealthy, exploitative or abusive by at least one of the partners. This is especially the case where the treatment of the other as object, rather than empathic caring, underlies the relationship. Masochistic elements may keep people in relationships that they experience in this way, because they feel they deserve to be treated badly, or because they fear the consequences of refusing to go along with their partner's wishes. Such people may also consent to more ordinary sexual activities against their feelings, for the same reasons.

Emotional immaturity expressed through partner choice

In looking at the ideas put forward by Dicks (1967) in Chapter 3, we saw how choice of partner can be an attempt to solve earlier difficulties, and how connections between partner choice and unconscious needs have consequences for the kind of sexual relationship and sexual difficulties that emerge. We noted that this may be helpful if such difficulties are not too great; 'if the marriage provides a container in which the partners give each other enough time, space and trust to enable them to work through their shared level of disturbance' (Daniell 1985: 173). Balint (1993: 41–2) says that 'in marriage we unconsciously hope to find a solution to our intimate and primitive problems, particularly to those which we feel we cannot communicate socially in an acceptable way'. The mechanisms by which this operates are elaborated by Lyons, who says that

> the unconscious drive to individuate leads people to choose partners who will activate undeveloped parts of themselves. This may lead sometimes to marrying a partner who resembles the parent who originally 'had it all'. Such an idealized choice offers a path on the one hand to individuation, and on the other to a source of continuing envy.
>
> (Lyons 1993: 48)

Particularly pertinent in heterosexual attraction is the relevance of the relationship to the opposite-gender parent (or other significant adults of the opposite sex during childhood), or the absence of any such figure. In homosexual attraction we might expect the same-sex parent to perform a similar role. Idealization of such a significant person is likely to lead to the choice of a similar person for a partner. On the other hand, choices can sometimes seem to be a reaction against someone seen as a 'bad' parent, where the person is attracted to someone with apparently opposite characteristics. Frequently people select a partner whose underlying personality resembles that of a significant other. This often turns out to be the case even when the choice is of someone who at first appears to be quite different. These kinds of parental transferences onto a partner may arouse incestuous anxieties resulting in such difficulties as loss of interest of sex for women, or erectile dysfunction for men. A man might choose a woman to meet his mothering needs, but then find that he cannot obtain an erection when making love to her because of incestuous anxieties.

Pincus and Dare quote from an unpublished manuscript by Lyons:

> Any man whose awareness of women still refers directly to his experience of his mother, and who has not been able to

see relations with other women as a symbolic, and therefore acceptable, way of securing her for himself, suffers considerable inhibitions in his sexual life. In his unconscious
mind his wife is his mother, and his behaviour with his
spouse is inhibited by the taboo appropriate only to the idea
of having sexual relations with one's mother. It is common
for a couple to find that difficulties of this kind either first
appear or, if already present, become greatly exacerbated,
when the first child is born. The wife comes to share even
more properties and roles of the man's own mother, making
it harder still for him to distinguish between the original
object of his emotion and its present-day substitute.

(Pincus and Dare 1978: 57)

In other instances sexual problems may occur where immaturity is expressed through the construction of a parent–child
dynamics which again introduces anxiety-raising incestuous elements, or where unwanted projections produce hostility between
the couple. We look more specifically at such mechanisms as idealization and identification in the discussion that follows.

Problems associated with defence mechanisms

It is important to be aware that anxiety states, depression and
paranoid tendencies are common expressions of the operation of
defences. These can be very disruptive both of a couple's general
and sexual relationships, and of an individual's sexual functioning. In this section we draw on the schema of defence mechanisms devised by Bateman and Holmes (1995).

Primitive or immature defences

Narcissism
This term is used in many ways, but we use it to refer to those
who organize their life and experience around themselves as a
point of reference. Within a sexual relationship it leads to a desire
in the person for sex to meet their own need for gratification. It
is difficult or impossible for such people to take into account a
partner's needs, or partner's objections to agreeing to what is
experienced by them as unacceptable sexually. Not uncommonly
a man will be preoccupied with meeting his own sexual needs

and cannot empathize with his partner's disinterest. He cannot understand why there is a problem and why his partner will not just comply with his needs.

Splitting

The division of an object into 'good' and 'bad' is a pervasive phenomenon and can be seen in a number of ways in relation to sexuality. Relationships can be split into the 'good' emotional closeness and the 'bad' sexual relating. Commonly one partner will own all the need for emotional relating, and the other all the needs for sexual relating. The genitals can be split off from the rest of the body, or from the relationship, and experienced as bad. This can produce a situation where the person avoids sexuality by attempting to exclude it from the couple relationship, for example by preoccupations with childcare, work or tiredness.

Idealization

This is a process by which a person is experienced in a split-off way (as above), with anything that does not fit the ideal picture denied or ignored, so that idealization can be maintained. Temporary idealization is a normal part of the experience of falling in love and is likely to enhance sexual relations. However, where this persists, it can cause sexual difficulties, such as when a man idealizes his partner to the point where sex with her would be to defile her. Generally it is more common for men to idealize women in this way, and it can form part of an unconscious agreement to avoid sex, where the woman has lost interest and the man finds it hard to express his need for sex.

Introjection

This is an attempt to overcome separation anxiety by internalizing an object. Often the process comes to light when couples become parents, and realize that they have internalized their own parents' attitudes when parenting their new offspring. Introjects can also be somatized by being projected onto genitalia or in some other way into sexual activity. In this way the introjection of parents' disapproval of sex may be expressed through vaginismus or disinterest in sex. In particular, some women lose interest in sex after the perceived end of their childbearing, where they have introjected an image of being a mother that has no place for sex unconnected to the idea of procreation.

Projection

This involves attributing difficult and unacceptable feelings and impulses to others, rather than accepting them as part of oneself, and normally works against establishing and maintaining a good sexual relationship. Where the good parts of the self are projected onto the other, the resulting increased feelings of lack of self-esteem are generally helpful. However, where negative aspects are projected, this can lead to avoidance of sex as an attempt to avoid the projected aspect. For example, someone may accuse their partner of continually starting an argument in a situation, where in fact they are themselves being provocative. They may then say that they do not feel like having sex with their partner while the partner is being so difficult.

Projective identification

We have seen how Klein's theory of projective identification suggests a phantasy through which the bad parts of the self are split off and projected into someone else, who is then experienced as the 'bad' parts of oneself. Theorists such as Spillius and Sandler use the term more widely to refer to a mutual process in which the projector and recipient interact with one another at an unconscious level. Similar potentials exist for the disruption of sexual relating as those arising from projection, for example as a defence to disown the sexual parts of the self.

Neurotic defences

Denial

This describes the refusal to acknowledge that there is a problem, commonly used by one partner in a couple relationship when they need to avoid facing a particular situation. One person may complain that sex only happens every few months, while the partner cannot see this as a problem, even though it is clearly causing distress for the partner.

Dissociation

This device is often used in a sexual relationship where a person does not want to take part. Sex becomes an experience where the person feels distance or uninvolved, or even as if it is happening to someone else. This is not uncommon in people who have been sexually abused as children, and have used dissociation to cope with this. As adults the way they deal with sex is similar.

Often they describe watching themselves from above, or not having any recollection of what takes place during sex. They often deny having any sexual needs, in order to avoid getting in touch with difficult feelings and memories that have been repressed.

Identification

This term is used in a number of ways, for example to refer to the extension of a person's identity into someone else, or to describe the borrowing of identity from someone else. It involves some fusion of identity with another and is a normal part of the process by which self-representations are built up within a person. Some degree of identification is necessary for a satisfactory sexual relationship, but over-identification can be disruptive of an individual's autonomy. Anxiety about over-identification may lead, for example, to the avoidance of intercourse or the suppression of orgasm.

Intellectualization

Intellectualization is frequently encountered in counselling and therapy. Some clients resist getting in touch with their feelings and experience by talking in a cerebral way. Others habitually steer the sessions towards abstract considerations and avoid more intimate discussion. In sessions such clients often want to talk in technical terms or ask questions about the counsellor's work with other clients with the same problems.

Rationalization

This is another process commonly observed in work with clients. They offer logical and believable explanations for irrational behaviour that can clearly be seen to have been prompted by unconscious wishes. A common example is where clients explain carefully why they cannot find the time for sexual activity, whereas it is clear to the counsellor that a minor adjustment of priorities would solve the difficulty.

Reaction formation

This is the adoption of a psychological attitude diametrically opposed to a conscious wish or desire, and may happen where sexual interest arouses too much anxiety. Therefore some clients who express no interest in sex at all experience a radical change once their anxieties have been overcome.

Regression

It is inevitable that regression will take place in couple relationships. Part of their value is that this can be a safe place, where this can be allowed to happen. Most people regress to some extent during sexual activity. Where, however, it leads to overdependence, or the uncontrolled expression of problem emotions, it mitigates against good sex. Some couples seem to take turns in looking after each other, whereas in other relationships one has the clear role of carer. In other relationships one partner contains an extreme amount of anxiety or anger and seeks to help and protect the other at all times. Sex is a low priority in most regressed parent–child relationships.

Repression

Where anxieties and other negative feelings surround sexual material from early life, this is often removed from consciousness. Such repressed memories can interfere with adult sexual functioning, for example through flashbacks, if repression begins to fail. The idea of memories of sexual abuse being repressed and later recovered has created considerable controversy in recent years (e.g. Campbell 1995; Pop and Hudson 1995). It is important that counsellors and therapists do not act in ways that suggest sexual abuse where the client has not spoken of this possibility, and that they follow the guidelines that have been produced in the wake of this controversy (UKCP 1997).

Reversal

In this defence there is a movement to the opposite of what is actually being felt. This is very close to the idea of reaction formation, from which it is not always clearly distinguished. In general it can be said that in reaction formation there is a tendency to exaggerate the opposite, whereas in reversal there is a move away from an active reaction towards a passive one. For example, someone with a high level of sexual interest who fears the consequences of being sexually demanding may adopt a sexually passive stance.

Somatization

This is particularly applicable to sexual difficulties because it involves the projection of a problem onto the body. Thus Eichenbaum and Orbach describe how somatized phobias such as vaginismus after marriage can be triggered by loving relationships:

Such a relationship may be psychically disconcerting if it is in strong contrast with what a woman has become habituated to. She may have longed for a close relationship but be overwhelmed by its actuality because it brings up all the hidden feelings of rage, loss and hurt caused by disappointment with her original love object, and it exposes the hidden little-girl. If the woman cannot contain these feelings they become somatized.

(Eichenbaum and Orbach 1985: 165–6)

They see vaginismus as a symptom that illustrates the somatization of boundary problems in a particularly clear way:

One way to understand vaginismus is to see it as expressing a woman's fear of being taken over, of being invaded and losing herself. Having a shaky sense of her psychological boundaries, she must protect the only boundary she knows, her physical body . . . The rigid boundaries expressed through the closing of the vagina prevent merger because merger means disintegration and loss of self in the other.

(p. 166)

Mature defences

Such defences allow the partial expression of underlying wishes and desires, but in a socially acceptable way. People may use *humour* as a way of dealing with sexual difficulties. This can be a feature in sessions with clients where interventions are blunted or discounted by humour, and the therapeutic process diverted. In other instances it is clear that sexual interest and energy is being *sublimated*, perhaps into a parental role where a couple show great passion about caring for their children, but little romantic or sexual desire for each other.

Exploring sexual problems in terms of family dynamics

With the birth of children most relationships move from a dyadic intimate world to a more complicated multi-person situation. The dynamics involved in this shift take people some time to get used to. Even where the original dyad does not survive because of separation, families contain numbers of individuals who are related, but not necessarily living together all the time. Thus family life tends to be fluid and punctuated by the composition of different styles of relationship throughout its life cycle. Not all relationships are the same, and not all psychodynamic processes that occur in relationships produce difficulties such as sexual problems. However, the circumstances and behaviour of other family members can sometimes play a part in the development of sexual symptoms, as the following case study illustrates.

> Rod came to the clinic alone, saying that his wife was to busy to attend. He had been married for 28 years and had two sons, one of whom was currently living at home. Rod worked as a taxi driver at night, which meant that sex with his partner used to take place during the day. Three years previously, at the age of 55, he had noticed that his erections were collapsing each time he attempted to make love to his wife. They both thought that the problem was related to his age, and started to avoid sex. However, Rod had come to feel miserable at the loss of his sex life, and had decided to try and sort his problems out. He sent away for information about sexual problems, in response to adverts in magazines, but this had no beneficial effect. We discussed his family and he was asked about any stressful events that may have occurred. The son at home was a drug addict who was currently waiting for a bed in a rehabilitation unit. Rod described the nightmare of events that had unfolded over the last five years since his son had admitted his drug problem. He could no longer trust his son, who had stolen from him, and felt angry that he and his wife could not agree on how to deal with the problems generated by the son living with them. As a result he had washed his hands of the situation. He had come to feel impotent in this situation, and excluded from the very intense relationship between mother and son.
>
> The second interview included his wife, who made it very clear that her priority was her adult son, and that she did not want to come for any psychological help. Rod continued to come to therapy, dealing with the anger, disappointment and feelings of powerlessness that were undermining him. He was encouraged to interpret his sexual symptoms as part and parcel of what was happening within the family. Despite washing his hands of his son he was still deeply upset by the situation and directly affected by his son's behaviour. His inability to deal with how he felt or to affect any significant changes in his

son's life left him denying his deep upset. His exclusion from a sexual relationship with his wife was a tangible sign of the general exclusion that he felt within the family. To an extent he was unconsciously jealous of his son, fearing that his partner no longer needed him and that she had replaced him with their son. Her lack of interest in sex unconsciously confirmed this to him. He was encouraged to make explicit his sexual and emotional needs with his partner, and to assert his need to be part of the couple, separate from their concerns as parents.

He also worked with memories from his childhood. Rod was the middle child of three born to a coal miner and his wife. His childhood was full of envious and guilty feelings that he had towards his brother who was a year younger than him, and had been born with cerebral palsy. He connected this to his current feelings about his wife and son, and realized that in a similar way he was feeling envious towards his son. In a sense the nightmare for Rod was about dealing with feeling replaced and unloved, and finding some way to resolve these feelings. Marrying someone who made him feel like 'a million dollars' meant that he had successfully avoided this unresolved situation until family circumstances had changed.

Unconscious processes of projection, denial and projective identification enable a couple to displace their anxieties. This does not deny the importance of the reality of external events and their effect on family life. However, balancing the needs of the different individuals requires that couples do not lose sight of their own relationship, which needs to survive while it contains the comings and goings of other family members, the arrival and departure of children, the development and aspirations of the individuals, as well as illness and eventual death of one partner. These and other issues can be points at which defensive processes operating within the family no longer contain difficulties.

Sexuality in the transference and countertransference

In psychodynamic sex therapy the information communicated through the transference forms part of the unconscious processes that underlie therapy. The transference will contain something of the dynamics between the couple, as well as information about both individuals' internal emotional worlds, and the unconscious process between clients and therapist. Sexuality and desire can be acted out in the transference through disowning and projecting of sexual thoughts and impulses. Erotic, dangerous and idealized thoughts and feelings can take the shape of intense feelings directed towards the therapist. The discussion of erotic material increases the risk for both therapists and clients that they might act on their feelings, instead of containing them. A highly sexualized transference may be narcissistically gratifying for the clinician, and may be colluded with, instead of being thought about, in terms of what is really being communicated. 'It can be flattering to be idealised and exciting to be the object of intense desire' (Maguire 1995: 137). In this way therapists may deny their own seductive behaviour and not make the kind of transference interpretations which will enable the client to move forward.

Maguire (1995) further points out how defences against change exhibited through the transference need to be thought about, although traditionally there has been a gender imbalance in this discourse. Most reports are of female clients falling in love with their male therapist, yet sexualized transferences from male clients to female therapists do happen, as do same-sex transferences. This gender bias of the transference needs careful analysis, as does the maternal transference of the male client to the female therapist, which may be just as erotic. Maguire argues that there are cultural and psychic reasons for this under-reporting, including therapists' unconscious anxieties and conflicts, all of which affect the ability to analyse the countertransference. Gender issues of sexuality and authority are also involved. Sex therapists have to work with the interface between unconscious and conscious erotic fantasy and reality. Within the area of perversions the needs for clients to humiliate, dominate and subjugate either themselves or others can reveal itself through the psychodynamic processes of the transference.

> James presented to the sex therapy clinic with what he described as a compulsive need to visit prostitutes. During his visit he would ask them to insert chocolate into his anus to simulate defecation, and it was only during this activity that he was able to be sexually aroused and able to achieve an erection. Consequently forming sexual relationships with non-prostitutes was difficult, as women reacted with disgust when he made such requests. During

supervision the therapist became increasingly aware of her countertransference reactions of frustration, anger, and feeling used. It was suggested that perhaps she was being used in a similar way to the prostitutes, and that James was unable to acknowledge anger, and needed help to process his feelings and thoughts. It was suggested that it was as if the therapist was being unconsciously asked to bear James's anger. His preoccupation with his anus and what he produced was connected to his unresolved Oedipal issues towards his mother, and these were being re-enacted through his relationship with the prostitutes and the therapist.

Conclusion

This chapter has explored the main psychodynamic concepts relevant to understanding and working with people who have sexual difficulties. We have noted that a psychodynamic approach does not have to be used exclusively. The ability of the therapist to be able to use the psychodynamic approach with a particular client depends not just on an understanding of the process and its relevance to the presenting problem, but also an ability to assess the extent to which the client will be able to benefit from such an approach. Any assessment of a client's difficulties needs to include an understanding of the limits of a purely psychodynamic approach, such as the need for physical therapy as part of the treatment. Within the sex therapy field it is now widely acknowledged that the way forward is a more comprehensive provision of services for people with sexual difficulties, which includes the psychodynamic alongside behavioural, systemic and medical perspectives (Riley 1998). We now turn in the final two chapters to the more practical aspects of the assessment and treatment of sexual problems.

Chapter 5

General and psychodynamic aspects of the assessment of sexual problems

In assessing clients for psychodynamic work with sexual difficulties it is important also fully to address the kind of general issues that would be relevant in using *any* therapeutic approach. These include medical and psychiatric issues, sex and gender, age, race and ethnicity. For many clients the initial difficulty is talking explicitly about sex, and it is to this issue we turn first.

Talking about sex

There are many reasons why it is a big step for some people to begin to discuss a sexual problem (see Table 5.1). While social attitudes about talking about sex have changed over the last thirty years, the subject is still fraught with difficulties, and consequently people vary in their degree of ease in talking about sexual problems. Many couples find it hard to talk to each other, and some find it easier to reveal the extent of their difficulty to a professional than to their partner. Others cannot talk to anyone about such an intimate area of their lives, or see such a discussion as a threatening invasion of their privacy. For these and other reasons people often tolerate problems for many years before seeking help or even mentioning it to someone who might be able to advise them. Some clients already in counselling, or who have had previous psychological help, talk about all kinds of intimate and difficult material, and yet are still reluctant to discuss sexual issues. While many people have the confidence and ability to talk about their problem directly, others say nothing about their sexuality unless they are led gently towards the subject, or asked about it, although they may approach the subject indirectly, or drop 'hints' to see whether the counsellor follows up what they say. Comments that might be made include:-

'My husband and I are arguing all the time nowadays.'
'He just can't manage it like he used to.'
'I wish he would not keep bothering me while I am feeling so ill.'
'She does not seem interested in me at the moment.'
'We have found it best to sleep in separate beds since I came out of hospital.'
'We just don't seem to be getting on so well since my operation.'
'Things haven't been the same between us recently.'

Such statements are so vague that they could mean many things. But one possibility is that there is some kind of sexual problem that the person would like to talk about.

The difficulty in discussing sexual matters sometimes results from people not being sure what words to use. Should they use 'medical' ones which they are not confident that they can pronounce correctly, or more familiar ones that may offend? If they get into difficulties they may be unsure whether the counsellor will help them out, or whether they will be left to stumble and so become even more uncomfortable. In generic counselling clients may also be worried that the counsellor will be embarrassed or uneasy if they broach the subject of sex. They may be

Table 5.1 Talking about sex – reasons clients find it difficult

- cultural norms and beliefs about sexuality, e.g. 'This is what I must expect at my age.'
- embarrassment
- exposure of difference from other people
- invasion of privacy
- lack of vocabulary
- past experiences in medical settings put them off taking further risks
- worry that nothing can be done
- worry that the problem will not be taken seriously

confident that counsellors are able to talk about many problem situations, but not sure that this includes sexual matters. In resolving these difficulties Hawton (1985: 103) helpfully advises that counsellors should

> find out what terms the partners understand, and then try to reach some common ground over the vocabulary to be used in the future. Some terms, such as 'to come' describing either a man's ejaculation or a woman's orgasm, are almost universally used by lay people and can usefully be employed in treatment.

Enabling clients to use their own terminology to describe their difficulties, as Hawton suggests, is a useful strategy, and may also give indications about how much clients understand sexual functioning as well as how far they are at ease in discussing sexual matters. The use of correct medical and diagnostic terminology by the therapist and client should be viewed with caution, since it may be based on the assumption of a shared understanding that does not exist in reality.

It is not unusual for clients to have consulted other practitioners, or to have read about their problems in popular newspapers and magazines before they eventually seek psychotherapeutic help. This in itself has an effect on language and thinking about such problems. As Dallos and Dallos (1997: 5) point out, 'it is hard to ignore the barrage of information about sex; how to do it, how to make it more satisfying, how often is normal, and what to do about it'. They suggest that such advice can often contain 'many unsupported assumptions about the nature of sexuality' (p. 3). The context within which clients are seen inevitably has an influence on how they and their therapists approach sexual problems, especially at the initial assessment session. For example, in NHS clinics for sexual and relationship problems some clients attend without undue anxiety about focusing on intimate sexual matters because this is what they expect. Their concerns may be more about the outcome of the interview and whether they are going to obtain help, especially if they have long-standing difficulties. It is important, therefore, not to make assumptions about the degree of difficulty that clients may have in talking about such intimate areas of their lives. Table 5.2 raises questions about the counselling context that practitioners might further wish to consider.

Table 5.2   Talking about sex – some questions to consider

- If one of your clients wants to talk about a sexual problem with you, how easy is it for them?
- What is your reaction to them?
- Are there any specific things that might put them off?
- What changes to your approach and technique might make it easier for people to talk about their sexual problems?

Medical and psychiatric issues in assessment

Medical and psychiatric issues are important considerations both in assessment and ongoing counselling. Chronic illness is usually an unforeseen and unwanted process of change to which adjustment needs to be made; for some, an important part of this adjustment is the accommodation of sexual or relationship problems. Difficulties in the sexual relationship may for some couples seem trivial in the light of their illness, but for others sexual physical closeness takes on a new importance and they are keen to obtain help with any problems. Where a sexual difficulty has a physical cause that cannot be removed or alleviated, the counsellor may need to help clients accept that they have to modify their goals in response to their illness or disability. This involves enabling them to deal with their reactions to changes that have been imposed and are resented, facilitating the acceptance of aspects that cannot be changed, and helping them to come to terms with loss (Jones *et al.* 1995).

It is not surprising that health challenges sometimes threaten the stability of close relationships. There is evidence that the rate of break-up of relationships may double in the face of seriously chronic health problems. However, there is also evidence that through periods of illness some relationships can be preserved, effectively restructured, or even improved. Most research in this area has been carried out in relation to neurological and vascular illness and disability, and there is a need for additional research that will identify specific interventions in close relationships that improve coping in illness (see Jones *et al.* 1995). A wide variety of both acute and chronic illnesses affect sexuality. In some instances a sexual problem may be the first identifiable symptom of a serious physical condition requiring treatment. For example, in a significant number of cases an erectile problem in men is the first symptom of diabetes, or it can be an early indicator of general vascular disease associated with heavy smoking. Minor acute illnesses such as colds and flu often have an impact on sexual interest, although such effects are normally temporary. In major acute episodes the inevitable disruption of sexual interest and functioning is normally overshadowed by more pressing considerations. The sexual problems associated with chronic illness can be divided into two categories: those that are likely to be associated with any chronic illness (Table 5.3), and those that arise from particular conditions (Table 5.4). The main problems likely to be associated with any chronic illness are lowering of libido, or difficulties in arousal, or (not uncommonly) both. The physical routes through which these operate are listed in Table 5.5.

Integrating physical assessments with the psychological assessment

During the assessment of psychosexual difficulties it is important that clients have access to medical assessment when needed. Clients with worries about the physical appearance or other

Table 5.3 Possible causes of low libido or difficulties in arousal in chronic illness

- anxiety as a secondary psychological reaction to illness
- depression as a secondary psychological reaction to illness
- discomfort
- drug and treatment side-effects
- pain
- tiredness

Table 5.4 Main physical sources of sexual problems

- drug and treatment side-effects
- general vascular
- hormonal disorders
- local genito-urinary
- local vascular
- neurological
- psychiatric
- skeletal
- skin diseases
- surgery, especially in the genital area

Table 5.5 The physical routes through which chronic illness can interfere with sexual functioning

- general health, e.g. cardiovascular disease
- physical disruption of sexual interest, e.g. hormonal
- physical disruption of sexual arousal, e.g. erectile problems caused by diabetes
- mediated disruption of sexual interest and/or arousal, e.g. via pain or depression
- physical disruption of orgasm, e.g. drug effect on ejaculation
- effect on self-image, e.g. skin disease, mastectomy
- infection, e.g. genital warts
- mobility restriction, e.g. arthritis

aspects of their genitalia can benefit from an examination that hopefully either confirms or denies a rational basis for their concern. Generally a medical assessment will consist of a medical history-taking and, where indicated, physical examination and further investigations, such as blood tests. Erectile dysfunction is the most common presenting sexual problem where blood tests can be important, as they can detect diabetes, hormonal difficulties and thyroid problems. In specialist clinics erectile difficulties can be further assessed through the use of equipment that measures the blood flow into the penis, as well as the blood pressure and tumescence of the penis. Where there are organic problems the onset of the problem is generally gradual, and the man cannot obtain a satisfactory erection in any situation. Typically the man feels aroused but there is no physical response from his penis. Further discussion usually reveals the absence of nocturnal and early morning erections (which are not under conscious control, and are responses to REM sleep). Such absence is an indication of organic difficulties which need to be considered as part of the assessment process.

For women there are a more limited number of relevant physical investigations. Internal vaginal examinations are part of detecting the physical aetiology of pain, but often reveal nothing of significance. Historically many of these problems have been seen as some form of somatization, especially when nothing could be detected (McKay 1988). However, more recently it has been discovered that vulval discomfort can have a variety of identifiable causes, including dermatological skin conditions, and that the contributory factors can be multifaceted (Wylie *et al.* 1999). Physical investigations are certainly advisable if it is difficult to come to any clear understanding of the cause of a client's problem, and where clients are unshakeably convinced that there is a physical cause to be discovered.

In a multi-disciplinary team it is important for the team members to be clear about their various areas of expertise and responsibilities, and for this to be appropriately communicated to clients. For example, the interpretation of blood tests made by medical colleagues can be communicated to clients by psychodynamic therapists if the effect of such interventions upon the relationship with the client is taken into account.

> Adrian, a man of 50 with erectile problems, had a series of blood tests as part of his assessment. They all came back normal and he was visibly disappointed. Both he and his partner spoke of how undermined they felt, as they had convinced themselves that the problem was physical. A number of sessions were spent sorting out the implications of what had happened, and in carrying out a more thorough assessment of their difficulties. This resulted in them making a decision that they did not want currently to embark on counselling, but understood that it was a possibility for them at some future date.

It is important that non-medical counsellors and therapists do not embark on psychological treatments without medical issues being properly covered. This kind of medical input can be relatively easily arranged where clients are being seen within a medical setting, but it is more difficult for practitioners in other settings. Where a referral is from a GP, the counsellor hopes that medical causes have been excluded, but it is still important to refer back to the GP if the counsellor has concerns about physical causes. Where clients self-refer or come from a non-medical setting, practitioners should be wary of taking on clients presenting with a sexual problem without having suitable medical cover. In particular, counsellors need to be careful in relation to sexual difficulties that may be the first symptom of serious physical illness, such as erectile problems in relation to diabetes. Even experienced counsellors and therapists should not work independently without access to medical consultation. It is important to remember that the presence of an organic abnormality does not necessarily identify the main or only cause of the sexual symptom (Riley 1998).

Counsellors whose normal practice is not to take notes in

the sessions should consider doing so when this is needed to establish a clear record of medical details, such as current medication and previous medical procedures, or where a history is very complicated. More information on medical and psychiatric issues can be found in texts such as Bancroft (1989) *Human Sexuality and its Problems* and Daines *et al.* (1997) *Medical and Psychiatric Issues in Counselling*. The psychodynamic practitioner also needs to take the meanings of any investigations, and the part played by other health professionals, into the work with clients as part of the transferential situation and as what has been termed the 'therapeutic triangle'. This is illustrated by the case example of Joseph.

> Joseph, a young man in his twenties, presented to the psychosexual clinic complaining of difficulties in achieving an erection. This problem emerged over a five-year period during which he felt powerless in the face of the difficulties that confronted him. His father, whom he described as 'the best dad ever', had died four years previously. He saw his mother occasionally, although it was never sufficiently often to satisfy her. Joseph came to feel torn between his mother and his girlfriend, feeling guilty that he did not spend enough time with his mother, and guilty that he was not able to satisfy his girlfriend sexually. The assessment generated enough information for the therapist to formulate Joseph's problems in terms of some very clear unresolved Oedipal dilemmas. His idealized relationship with his father and ambivalent relationship with his mother (and his partner) suggested incomplete separation and individuation processes.
>
> During the assessment Joseph requested a physical assessment of his erectile difficulties as he was concerned that he had a physical problem that was being ignored. Despite the therapist's reassurances that his history did not suggest any physical problems, it was clear that Joseph had his mind set on proceeding down this path. After about six sessions Joseph's appointment for the physical tests arrived, the results confirming the initial assessment that there was no evidence of an organic problem. However, Joseph's reaction to the male doctor and the tests was quite revealing. He described feeling humiliated by the investigations, and embarrassed by the doctor's presence. It reminded him of feeling guilty about touching his genitals

at the age of 14. He was angry with the doctor that he had been put through the tests and regretted that he had not listened to the female therapist's reassurances. This reaction was used to help Joseph look at his idealized relationship with his father, who he felt had ultimately let him down by dying. In a similar way the male doctor had been idealized as holding the answers to his problems, but had then let him down by 'making' him feel so awful. Joseph was precipitated into looking more closely at his relationship with his father, and this led to mourning not only his loss through death, but also the loss of the perfect image of a father who had in fact been quite a distant and unavailable figure in his childhood.

The relationship between chronic illness and couple relationship problems is described in Table 5.6.

The next example describes relationship difficulties existing alongside a physically caused sexual problem.

Alan and Moira, a couple in their late forties, went to their GP concerned about Alan's increased difficulties in achieving an erection. After a number of consultations and investigations it was established that he had arterial damage in his penis as a result of his long-standing

Table 5.6 The impact of chronic illness on couple relationships

Chronic illness can have a fundamental impact on couple relationships and the consequent problems can have a knock-on effect on the couple's sexual relationship (Jones *et al.* 1995). Such problems include:

- the disruption of the couple's normal pattern of activities together
- the exacerbation of existing difficulties
- the generation of negative emotions within the relationship, e.g. disappointment, frustration, envy, anger, fear, anxiety, insecurity, resentment
- infertility
- the interruption of an existing process of relationship breakdown
- maintaining communication, the need for which may have increased
- resolving difficulties and problems surrounding the illness
- role changes and disruption of previous dynamics in the relationship, e.g. power, dependency, responsibility
- specific difficulties associated with particular illnesses, e.g. communication difficulties following a stroke

insulin diabetic condition. A year or so later Moira visited the same GP because she was depressed. It transpired that she had been feeling isolated and lonely for quite a while, and was struggling to accept the lack of sexual activity in their relationship. They were referred to the local psycho-sexual clinic assessment and both attended for the initial session. During this session Moira remained fairly quiet, while Alan spoke at length about his erection difficulties and his diabetic condition. He seemed relieved to be able to talk about his situation and to share his conclusion that he could not see the situation improving. In contrast Moira hardly said a word or moved, except when agreeing with Alan about what the doctors had said. The counsel-lor commented on this, pointing out that she was aware that it was Moira who had initially gone to her GP for help. At this point Moira spoke of her own hopelessness about the situation, and said that she was sure that they were wasting the therapist's time.

Over the course of a number of consultations it became apparent that Moira felt rejected by Alan, and believed that his diabetes was a way of his avoiding any contact with her. In fact Moira commented that she thought Alan was more interested in his diabetes than he was in her. They both blamed the diabetes for their situa-tion, and were reluctant to try and find a way of still having some sexual contact in their relationship. Alan for his part realized that he had been avoiding any intimacy with her, because he no longer felt like a 'proper' man. During their therapy they became aware that they both had at different points in their relationship felt rejected by the other, and neither had addressed these feelings. When Alan became diabetic this situation carried on and they had grown further apart. By the time Alan started having erection difficulties they were rarely having any sexual contact, and were relieved that they did not have to try. All their anger and disappointment was projected onto the illness. It prevented them from having sexual contact, and at the same time served to protect them from each other's powerful feelings. It allowed them to carry on relating, although Moira's depressed state had brought their prob-lems to a head. With support and counselling they began to address their relationship difficulties, and the ways in which they could still be sexually active.

Gender issues

There are important gender differences surrounding seeking help. Women are usually more willing to ask for counselling and find it easier than men to talk about their problems. In contrast many men are more reluctant to see something as a problem, less aware of others' perception of their difficulties, and therefore less willing to consider going for help (O'Brien 1990). Where a problem is clearly perceived by men, they often present these as the result of their partner's difficulties, or insist that there is a physical cause, and do not see any need to attend as a couple. Faced with a physical sexual difficulty, they therefore often see no logic in the counsellor's interest in their relationship. Patterns of referral to sex and relationship clinics reveal gender differences in the kind of problem presented. Referrals of women typically focus on issues of desire and arousal: lack of sexual desire, loss of interest in sex, or not wanting sex as frequently as their partner. Conversely for men the problems presented tend to be about their performance: premature ejaculation, a variety of erection problems, and anxiety about their genitals. These gender differences reflect differing mental sets in recognizing problems. Men respond to the external signs concerning their genitals and the frequency of sex, whereas women are more concerned about feelings and the quality of the relationship (see Dallos and Dallos 1997: 154).

The gender of the therapist is also significant. Some clients have a clear preference and state it if given a choice at the pre-assessment enquiries. Obviously the therapist needs to bear this in mind, especially if the client's sexual experiences include any trauma. Ideally concerns surrounding the gender of a therapist should be identified by the referrer so that appropriate allocation can be made, but where this does not happen these issues can be resolved at assessment. However, in some instances these issues do not emerge until counselling is established, and then need to be addressed within that context. Even when such preferences can be accommodated, it is important to use this information as part of understanding the possible psychodynamics underlying clients' problems.

Age issues

Sexuality in our society tends to be seen as belonging to the young. 'There is a general expectation that normal ageing includes a dissipating sexual response, so that what is seen as normal sexuality at one age becomes sexual deviance at another' (Power-Smith 1984: 1). Thus the elderly in our society tend not to be viewed as sexual or encouraged to continue sexual activity. In fact their sexual behaviour is often ignored or pathologized (Power-Smith 1992). Sandford (1983: 46) suggests that the adjustment to ageing in relation to sexuality involves acknowledgement of the changes that are occurring, and an acceptance that they are inevitable. Once there is an understanding of what is happening and why, then both mental and physical adjustments can be made. While younger counsellors may need to address their attitudes to older clients, older counsellors may need to examine their reactions of disapproval to some of the activities of the young who come to them for help. It can be particularly difficult if clients are of an age similar to either the therapist's parents or children.

Ethnicity and sexuality

Working psychosexually across cultures is affected particularly by the existence of different belief systems about sexuality and sexual practices, as well as by customs and religion (Petrak and Keane 1998: 13–17). It is important to be aware of such relevant cultural knowledge, although this alone is not sufficient. Counsellors need also to be critically aware of their own attitudes and expectations, together with those of their clients. We must not assume that we are free from the effects of the racism that informs ethnic stereotypes and projections, and which can distort our understanding of the sexual problems presented by clients from different cultures. Being critically aware of such prejudice enables us to question the assumptions that underlie stereotypes, rather than act upon them. D'Ardenne and Mahtani (1989: 81–2) note that therapists' attitudes and expectations can be as much of a difficulty as those of the client from another culture.

For example, where counsellors have low expectations of their clients' success, these may affect the outcome of therapy. Lorion and Parron (1985) present evidence that clients from different ethnic groups find it hard to become established in counselling, and often terminate earlier than other clients. It is often assumed that this is due to these clients' expectations, such as the need to medicalize problems, the desire for a quick cure, a lack of verbal skills, and an unwillingness to form therapeutic relationships. However, the authors quote several studies showing a correlation between counsellors who have low expectations of success with ethnic clients and who anticipate a poor outcome in counselling. As a minimum D'Ardenne and Mahtani (1989: 36–41) suggest that we need to be very careful in assessing our own beliefs about counselling when we start working with a client from another culture. It is easy to blame the client (or for the client to blame themselves) for lack of success, when the problems lie elsewhere.

Psychodynamic assessment of sexual difficulties

Treating sexual problems from a psychodynamic perspective may arise as a possibility either when such a difficulty emerges in ongoing work or a result of a referral or a specific sexual problem. In either case a careful and comprehensive assessment has to be made that does not view the presenting sexual problem in isolation. The purpose of the assessment is to gain a reliable understanding of the genesis, development and maintenance of the problem, and to come to a conclusion about how it might be resolved. This includes decisions about whether to work with the individual or the couple, and whether the sexual problem or wider issues (such as the relationship) need to be the focus of the counselling. In dealing both with couples and with individuals who have an established partner, it is particularly important to consider the relationship between the sexual and the general aspects of the relationship. Sexual problems can exist in the context of a good relationship, or be the manifestation of individual or couple difficulties. Of crucial importance is a consideration of any coexisting health issues, both physical and psychological. Alongside these it is also important to consider other major life events that may influence sexual functioning. A germane example is pregnancy, where alongside the effect on sexual interest and potential practical difficulties in lovemaking, the therapy itself may well be at risk of disruption, especially if the pregnancy is in an advanced stage. Unless the need for help is urgent, it is often better to postpone counselling until three to six months after the birth, when both sexual interest and life generally will have had a chance to settle down.

A useful overview of assessment is given by Hawton (1985), although he primarily considers assessment as a preliminary to sex therapy that is basically behavioural in approach. From the basic areas of assessment that he identifies we have developed a schedule that will enable the therapist to formulate the difficulties psychodynamically (see Tables 5.7, 5.8 and 5.9). In a psychodynamic assessment of a sexual problem it is important to give attention to aspects that may reveal information about unconscious processes. Taking a history in the areas suggested should enable the practitioner to form a hypothesis about the psychodynamics underlying the problem. Hopefully it will be possible to identify the unconscious factors in a client's partner choice, for example whether problems with the parent of the opposite sex are being repeated in the current relationship. It is particularly important to identify the main defences that could

Table 5.7 The psychodynamic assessment of sexual difficulties

- the nature and development of the sexual problem
  how have the client(s) come to this understanding
  why help is being sought now
- family background and parenting
- sexual experiences
  earliest memories and their effect
  start of sexual activity
- sexual education and sources of information
  important influences, including religious belief, and cultural norms
- the history of any previous and current relationships
  including any difficulties in other relationships
- the nature of any relationship problems/difficulties
- general health and any previous help for emotional/psychological
  difficulties
- use of alcohol and drugs, especially prescribed medication and
  history of smoking behaviour
- expectations of themselves and of the therapeutic help

N.b. the order in which this information is gathered and the number of sessions over which this happens needs to be adapted to fit in with particular clients and work settings.

Table 5.8 Unconscious processes in the assessment

- the non-verbal communication from the individual or couple
- the kinds of meanings that are attributed, particularly to sexual
  matters
- what is not said or appears to be avoided
- struggles that may indicate areas of resistance
- evidence of the nature of the transference
- the counsellor's countertransference

Table 5.9 Psychodynamic understandings of common presenting sexual problems

Sexual problems in women
- impaired sexual interest
  narcissistic partner
  projection
  projective identification
  dissociation
  regression
- lack of arousal
  dissociation
  repression
- orgasmic dysfunction
  schizoid fears
  denial
  repression
- vaginismus
  somatization, split off difficult feelings and thoughts
- dyspareunia including vulval pain
  usually physical, though can include somatization
- sexual phobias
  projection

Sexual problems in men
- erectile dysfunction
  identification
  somatization
  idealization
  sexual object choice
- premature ejaculation
  idealization
  expression of hostility
- retarded and non-ejaculation
  projection
  denial of ambivalence
- impaired sexual interest
  intellectualization
  projection
- sexual phobias
  projection
- pain
  somatization

Sexual problems manifesting primarily in a relationship
- differences of interest in sex
  conflict between need to merge and to differentiate
  projections and splitting of sexual interest
- difficulties in communicating about sex
  over-differentiation
  identification
- a general relationship difficulty causing a sexual problem
  projection onto sexuality
  shared emotional immaturity

---

underlie the sexual difficulty, or the kind of defence that the sexual problem itself represents. The role of defences is discussed in detail in the next chapter.

It is usual first of all to establish the nature of the sexual problem or dissatisfaction and, where this is difficult to do, to try to identify why this might be the case. Sometimes a number of related difficulties, such as depression, become intertwined with the sexual problem. Where this occurs it is necessary to assess how far it is possible to work on these more general psychological difficulties alongside the specific sexual problem, or whether these might have to be addressed first. Alternatively, the sexual difficulty may be secondary to relationship problems; it is not uncommon for couples to present with a sexual problem, and then to go on and describe serious underlying difficulties in their general relationship. An issue on which counsellors disagree is whether it is valid to run separate individual and conjoint work with different counsellors at the same time. Psychodynamic theory suggests that this should be avoided, because of the potential for various kinds of acting out, such as material generated in one situation being taken to the other. It can also be argued that confusion over transferences is created, and is difficult to resolve. From a pragmatic point of view, however, it appears unreasonable to expect an individual to have to terminate their individual counselling to try to save their relationship. A similar dilemma may face someone in couple therapy who urgently needs individual help. On balance we believe that the two can work successfully together, as long as the material belonging to each situation can be clearly delineated, and where both counsellors and clients are able to be disciplined about maintaining the appropriate boundaries between the two.

Jan and Sue presented to the local psychosexual clinic complaining that their lovemaking had become unsatisfactory. They explained how they had been living together for the last twenty years, and that during this time sex had generally been mutually satisfying. However, over the last two years they had both become uninterested and wondered whether they needed to learn new techniques, or whether the problems were associated with ageing. Both appeared to be happy with their relationship generally, and made light of their difficulties, perhaps hoping that some general reassurance or advice was all that was needed. It transpired during the next few sessions that, despite looking happy, Sue was deeply upset about a decision that 'they' took many years ago not to have children. She retained a fantasy that one day this decision would be altered, and that somehow her partner really did want a child, just like her. Of late she had struggled to maintain this fantasy, and become increasingly depressed as she began to develop ambivalent feelings towards her partner. In turn, her partner without realizing it, had reacted with irritation to this change. Together they had begun to focus on sex as the cause of their difficulties. Unconsciously they had colluded in avoiding the more serious issues that put their relationship in jeopardy.

In general it is better to conduct the first interview with the couple together, so that an assessment can be made of how far the problem is an individual difficulty or a couple problem, and whether it is best addressed by one or both of them attending future sessions. In our experience, couple dynamics can be pivotal, even when the presenting problem appears to be the result of clear organic factors. The ability of relationships to support, contain and facilitate adaptation to sexual dysfunction varies enormously, and may trigger secondary difficulties in the relationship. There is also evidence that a supportive relationship helps prognosis (Synder and Berg 1983; Baggaley *et al.* 1996). However, if for any reason it is considered important or essential to interview separately, it is better to do this on the understanding that the relevant content of these sessions can be incorporated into the couple counselling as necessary. In this way the practical and psychodynamic problems of 'secrets in the family' can be avoided. In particular the disclosure by one partner of an affair which they wish to keep secret can render the counsellor impotent, leaving them unable to work effectively with the sexual problems, and unable to explain to the partner who is in the dark why such work is not possible.

Research to compare outcomes of individual- and couple-orientated treatments for sexual and relationship problems has found significant differences (Hirst and Watson 1997). Whether a referral for a sexual problem is responded to by help for an individual or for the couple can affect the outcome. Hirst and Watson (1997) conclude that it is very important to assess the degree to which the problems presented are interpersonal, or particular to the individual, and to organize the therapy in accordance with this. However, the issue of whether the problem requires an individual- or couple-based approach is often prejudiced before clients attend for a first appointment by the views and actions of the referrer, or by the ideas of the clients themselves. Primary referrers, such as GPs, may not be trained to assess whether relationship difficulties underlie individual psychological or psychosomatic complaints (Burnap and Golden 1967; Rust *et al.* 1987). Further, Kayser (1993) points out that individuals who are in the early stages of relationship problems may not always be in a position to decide whether their problems need an individual or joint approach. Clearly all these issues need to be kept in mind by the therapist at the assessment stage.

It is important that sufficient time is taken to establish a reliable understanding of the problem, and of the best way to approach it. This generally takes between one and three sessions. In a generic counselling context, where there has been no initial presenting problem related to sexuality, clients may be anxious and unsure about the legitimacy or relevance of talking about such intimate parts of their lives. In such settings it is important to pace the work to make allowance for this. An assessment which extends to more than one session also allows time for a counsellor to obtain medical advice if necessary, and to discuss the situation in supervision before coming to a decision. It is helpful for clients to be given some explanation for the sexual difficulty as soon as possible, and to be told how this will guide treatment choice. In this way the formulation becomes part of the discussion held with clients in coming to an agreement about possible ongoing counselling. Where there are a number of possible areas of therapeutic work, this needs to be communicated to clients so that they can be involved in deciding whether there is going to be a wide scope to the counselling or whether to focus on a particular issue. The offer of help made may involve working towards

Table 5.10 Approaches to sexual problems

Cognitive/behavioural
- short/medium term
- the work is with the here-and-now
- the couple need to be able to comply with tasks set between sessions
- some degree of self-awareness is helpful

Systems
- usually short term
- useful for disorganized and complex relationships
- insight and compliance are not important

Psychodynamic
- medium/long term
- the couple need to be capable of self-awareness and able to work with insights
- they also need to see the relevance of the past for the present

Integrative
- generally short/medium term
- particular approach will often be tailored to needs of patients

---

a resolution, an alleviation or a means by which the difficulty might be better lived with.

One outcome might be the need to refer to someone offering a different kind of therapy. Within sex therapy there are currently three dominant approaches: cognitive-behavioural, systems and psychodynamic. Many people work with an integration of two of these but may also use aspects of other theories, such as transactional analysis. Key aspects of these main therapies are identified in Table 5.10. The decision to use one of these approaches or elements of different approaches is influenced not only by the assessment interview and the kind of material that is generated, but also by the availability of different approaches within the setting in which clients are being seen. At all points reassessment of the appropriateness and effectiveness of the approach used should form part of the counsellor's monitoring of the work and of discussion in supervision.

Conclusion

The decision to embark on psychodynamic work with an individual or couple presenting with a sexual difficulty must be undertaken only after a process of careful assessment, including medical and psychiatric aspects. In order to benefit from a psychodynamic approach there must be a preparedness by the clients to accept that the counselling is probably going to take between 10 and 20 sessions, and that it does not offer a quick solution to their difficulties. Furthermore, there needs to be a potential for self-awareness in clients and an ability to gain insight and relate this to their problems. Clients also need to be able to see the relevance of the past for the present, especially the crucial role of relevant childhood experiences. Proper assessment of sexual difficulties can take more than one session, especially if there is a complex mixture of medical and non-medical information to be processed. For the psychodynamic therapist information from the transference forms a pivotal aspect of their information-gathering. In all this it is important that therapists have adequate psychodynamic supervision, sources of medical advice and management support.

Chapter 6

Working psychodynamically with sexual problems

Moving from assessment to formulation

The main purpose of assessment is to arrive at some understanding of the problem, both in terms of causes and of possible ways of resolving it. The conclusion of this is a psychodynamic formulation, which is a working hypothesis that includes various aspects of the presenting problem, as well as historical and current references that may be contributing factors. On a practical level this summary serves as a check that the history-taking has taken account of the variety of influences outlined in the previous chapter. It demonstrates the interaction of physical, psychological and relational factors that could be contributing to the sexual problem, and enables the therapist to offer a rationale for the approach being offered.

Often when working with couples one of them is usually presented as the 'client', so that the formulation of the situation in terms of the couple relationship gives the therapist the opportunity to present a more balanced view. This can be achieved by highlighting aspects of the situation which resonate for both partners, and by helping them identify shared areas of difficulty. This 'couple perspective' aims to enhance understanding and tolerance of each other, pointing to their relationship as a possible focus, rather than one individual's difficulties alone. Not all couples find this shift easy to make, especially when one has had a medical assessment of the problems. However, the opposite can also be true inasmuch as the other can be relieved to be included.

As part of the formulation clients need to be offered a description of the current difficulty, and its possible relationship to present and past influences, perhaps unconscious as well as conscious. The language used should enable clients to identify themselves in the description offered (Lago and Thompson 1996) and avoid phrases that may be culturally incomprehensible. For example, an Afro-Caribbean woman asked her counsellor where the 'space' was located which was referred to during a session. Clients' responses to appropriate explanations offer an opportunity for the therapist to discuss the proposed approach, and for clients to make decisions about proceeding with further sessions.

> Celia and John attended for an assessment after a GP referral describing her difficulties with libido which had arisen post-operatively. She complained that she felt rarely sexual following a recent hysterectomy, and that her orgasms felt very different now. Celia believed that the operation had fundamentally affected her ability to feel sexual. She had discussed this with her doctor, who had dismissed her fears. Her partner was clearly angry, blaming the 'system' and complaining that the doctors were not prepared to help any further. They were concerned both that their relationship was suffering, and that she rarely felt like sex. The assessment was carried out over two sessions, ending with a formulation. The therapist suggested to the couple that there were two difficulties: one was Celia's ability to feel sexual and the associated problem with her orgasms, and the other was how as a couple they had experienced difficulties in response to these changes. The therapist hypothesized that Celia's change in her libido could be the result of a number of factors, including her experience that her orgasms now felt qualitatively different.
>
> One of the physical changes that might have affected Celia's experience was the removal of her uterus. For some women their orgasmic sensation is felt through the contraction of their uterus, and perhaps since the operation she was no longer able to experience this. The therapist suggested that there could also be other factors contributing to the difficulties. Celia described how she imagined that the operation had damaged her in some way, and this seemed to be confirmed by the way she now experienced herself sexually. The operation provoked and

somatized a variety of negative feelings and fantasies about internal damage and loss which left Celia feeling bad about what had happened to her body. They were both struggling with change, and experienced the help that they had received so far as ineffectual – as if someone was stopping them from getting what they needed.

It appeared that they both wanted their lives to stay the same, and yet the hysterectomy was forcing them to change. Without being aware of it, their protectiveness of each other was not helping to sort their difficulties out. In the same way their concentration on what had happened at the hospital, and how other people were letting them down, was not helping to resolve how they felt with each other. It seemed difficult for them to know how to deal with this problem with no further medical help on offer. Coming for a psychosexual appointment must have been difficult for them, as it was a second best. It implied a reluctant acceptance that further medical intervention was not going to happen. Additionally they were probably worried that the therapist would disappoint them. The therapist concluded the explanation by suggesting that perhaps Celia's libido problems were the result of a complex interaction of a number of factors, rather than any one thing, and that it was important to look at the meanings of what was happening and how these changes affected both of them and their relationship.

Initially this couple were sceptical about the value of working on their relationship, but stayed with it. Over a series of about 15 appointments they came to acknowledge and integrate some difficult feelings and thoughts that they had about each other. The sexual symptoms were accepted more, and integrated into the relationship. As a result less of their anger and disappointment needed to be projected onto the outside world. They discussed at length their early childhood experiences, realizing that they had each married someone whom they saw as an ideal, and that this was in some sense connected to their own experiences of idealizing their own parents. They both found conflict difficult, and up to this point had avoided ambivalent feelings towards each other by projecting 'disappointment' onto the outside world – doctors, hospitals and so on. Their mutual idealization was based on their unconscious wish to remain attached to their earlier family, and to retain the phantasy of the ideal parent. As such their difficulties presented them with an opportunity to make adjustments, and work through disappointment and disillusionment. This enabled them to have a more realistic relationship with each other, and with the outside world.

A proportion of clients presenting with sexual difficulties have already consulted with other health professionals about their problem. To varying degrees they will have already come to an opinion about whether the problem is physical or psychological. This often influences how they see the relevance of the approach to their problems. Resistance to working with problems in a more psychological way can be the result of seeing physical and psychological explanations as mutually exclusive, with the former perhaps being seen as in some way superior. However, there may also be deeper defensive and resistant processes operating within an individual. In order to help clients respond to the dynamic aspects of sexual difficulties any medical features need to be integrated into the formulation. Taking diabetes as an example, it is estimated that about 60 per cent of men with this disease have erectile difficulties, but it is clear that the degree of difficulty can vary enormously. In certain relationships the diabetes is blamed for everything, as it becomes the 'other' in the relationship, whereas in others it poses little difficulty despite its physical implications. Clearly there is a complex interrelationship between the various factors involved, leading to wide variations in individual and relationship dynamics. Working psychodynamically involves being able to hold this spectrum of information and understandings about diabetes, and considering what possible interpretations might be made.

One woman described how angry she was that every time she had a row with her husband he became ill and had to be hospitalized. Another described the visiting diabetic nurse as her husband's 'other woman' and felt excluded. In both these examples the illness altered the dynamics of a relationship to such an extent that the couples had ceased having a sexual relationship. Such couples find that the illness provokes change in their feelings towards each other. One of the women in an angry outburst put it this way: 'I feel I am being asked to be his mother, his nurse and occasionally his wife.' The diabetes was allowed to dominate both their lives, as disability and distance replaced sex and intimacy.

All these issues affect the formation of the therapeutic

alliance and the possibilities of creating a productive working relationship, which is essential if therapy is to proceed. Research into expectations of counselling has shown significant differences in the extent to which people perceive different approaches as credible or preferable (Shapiro 1981; Rokke *et al.* 1990). This suggests that therapists need to be more aware of how their clients perceive the help that is being offered. Though there is an absence of research into clients' perception of psychodynamic sex therapy we similarly need to check out how clients view this type of help. The evidence about time-limited therapy is that it is more effective when it matches client expectations (Morrison and Shapiro 1987; Hardy *et al.* 1995). The kind of formulation we have described is a working hypothesis that is inevitably tentative and needs to be modified at various points to take account of additional information that comes to light during later sessions. The counsellor should be wary both of sticking too long to a particular approach in the face of evidence to the contrary, but also of changing tack too soon or too often. Successful negotiation of the assessment phase and the initial formulation of sexual difficulties all form part of the beginning phase of psychodynamic work.

Individual and couple work

Having decided at the assessment to work either with the individual or the couple, it is common to feel a few sessions further on that the wrong decision has been made. There is a sense in which the problem always seems to be elsewhere, and this may be a consequence of the defences being employed. Working with a couple it is easy to become focused on the need for changes (in either or both of them) which would be more easily facilitated in individual counselling. Similarly, working with the individual, it can appear that the need for change is located primarily in the couple relationship. Clearly sometimes a wrong decision has been made at assessment, but it is best to wait a session or two, rather than make a change that later appears to have been unwise or premature. In individual work on sexual problems there is always a relationship component, even if the person does not currently have a partner. This may be in the form of unresolved issues and transferences from past relationships, or hopes or longings about possible future relationships.

In working with couples, it is important to recognize that

individual counselling skills are only partly transferable to couples work. Those who wish to offer couple counselling need specific training to understand the psychodynamics of the couple relationship, and to be able to work with these. Counsellors also need to adjust to working with a more dynamic situation where different kinds of interventions are needed to prevent domination by one partner, to deal with interruptions, and generally to ensure 'fair play'. This work can have a more organized agenda than individual work. It tends to be more practical and less abstract, partly as a result of the kind of regression being different from in individual work. However, in many ways the counselling situation is more complex, especially as there are three relationships in the room, rather than just one: client 1/client 2, client 1/counsellor and client 2/counsellor.

Co-therapy refers to a situation where two therapists work together as equals with a couple. A psychodynamic approach offers the clearest theoretical justification for co-therapy inasmuch as it involves the working-through of transference. It offers the opportunity for transferences related to each parent to be worked through for both partners. As projections and introjections are worked with in the transference towards both counsellors, they are withdrawn from the partner and a relationship less contaminated by the past can be built. For co-therapists to be able to work together well they need to be able to form a positive relationship with each other, and to be aware of and work through their own 'couple' issues, including their own transference onto the co-therapy partner. There are a number of general advantages that have been argued for co-therapy. One is that there is less likelihood that one of the couple is going to feel 'ganged up on' and without support in the session.

Assuming each partner in the couple has someone of the same sex in the co-therapy pair, each is more likely to feel supported on gender issues. Additionally one of the co-therapy pair can observe while the other talks. In this way the therapists can effectively support each other. However, there are no research findings that clearly demonstrate the effectiveness of two therapists over other therapy arrangements with couples. In fact the interest in and use of co-therapy has tended to decline in recent years because it takes over twice as much therapy time as the equivalent length of therapy offered by an individual, especially when the time for co-therapy planning and debrief is taken into account. Thus, although a case can be made out for co-therapy on theoretical grounds, its advantages are not proven.

Moving from formulation into therapeutic work

The formulation stage provides a guide as to the areas that need to be explored and worked through in actual therapeutic work. Scharff and Scharff (1991) usefully integrate Bion's concept of the container-contained and Winnicott's idea of the holding environment as a basis for this work with couples. They write that the 'relationship to the therapist creates a transitional space in which the couple can portray and reflect upon its current way of functioning, learn about and modify its projective identificatory system, and invent new ways of being' (Scharff and Scharff 1991: 108). The first task is to set the frame for counselling and to create psychological space. The expectation needs to be conveyed clearly that sessions will deal with the couple relationship, and not the two as individuals. Within firmly held boundaries the counsellor then listens to what the clients present, and allows their feelings to be expressed. It is important that the counsellor takes up a neutral position by maintaining a position described as 'involved impartiality'. This stance shows no preference to one partner or the other, to particular lifestyles, or to the outcome of treatment. The pressures to identify with one partner or to get distracted into the medical aspects of the problems are constant challenges. Containing the somatic and psychological aspects of the defence system can put the therapist under pressure as clients attempt to divert attention into unprofitable areas. Having good supervision and colleagues who can help hold and understand the impact of these different factors, provides essential support in working psychodynamically with individuals and couples, especially where there is a complex mixture of organic and psychological problems.

> Ron, a gay man with diabetes, was recovering from recent surgery for a cyst on his testes. The presenting problem was that he was unable to ejaculate and he had additionally been having bouts of depression for the last four years. It emerged that his parents had favoured his sister, and still as an adult actively supported her more than him. Ron was angry with them about this, and entertained the idea that his sister deserved more support than him. He rationalized this situation by projecting all his positive qualities onto his sister. His depression in turn protected him, by preventing him making any requests

for help from his parents, as well as from his partner, whom he feared would reject him. During the last four years he had been prescribed different types of anti-depressant medication. Discussion with a medical colleague revealed that his current medication had side-effects which included difficulties with ejaculation. This information enabled the client to seek a change in his medication, and to work more effectively on his sexual and emotional needs.

During therapy the counsellor tries to tune into the client's unconscious and to offer interpretations of the meanings of experiences. It is important to follow the themes that emerge from verbal associations, as well as to note and, where relevant, verbalize possible meanings of any silences. Counsellors can work with dream and fantasy material, and with unconscious communication expressed through physical sexual functioning. From this position the counsellor can offer interpretations of defences, anxieties, phantasies and inner object relations, and facilitate the working-through of the different issues. In looking at sexual problems in terms of defences it should be borne in mind that they overlap and interact and are not discrete, mutually exclusive categories.

As well as considering the psychodynamic causes of a difficulty, it is important also to explore introjected meanings which may be a consequence of the problems, e.g. 'It means I am not a real man' or 'I am an abnormal woman'. The therapist also actively encourages the use of the therapeutic relationship to contain the client's projections, and uses countertransference to make sense of projective processes. 'Through tolerating and then analysing our counter transference we can experience inside ourselves the couple's transference based on unconscious object relations' (Scharff and Scharff 1991: 83). Sometimes their countertransference is the most important tool available to the therapist.

After about a year's work with a man who had quite an unusual sexual practice, Jane noted how her feelings towards her client were becoming increasingly difficult to bear. As he described his need to hang himself by the neck during masturbation, she alternately felt anxious about him and angry towards him. During group supervision Jane described her difficulties and became aware of feeling very alone in the work, and somewhat abandoned by her colleagues. This facilitated the realization that her client's sexual behaviour had an important purpose as a distraction. The reality was that this man was struggling with feeling alone and abandoned, and possibly also with a deep sense of deprivation, and that the purpose of his sexual behaviour was to anaesthetize and dispel such problematic feelings. Through this process she was able to help the client understand his behaviour and reclaim and integrate the split-off projected parts of himself.

In time-limited work the therapist has to be more aware of how the time boundary may affect the client. The existence of a definite date for ending can have a variety of influences both on the individual and the couple, and may provoke anxiety in the therapist, especially if apparent progress is reversed towards the end of therapy.

A young couple, Tom and Beth, came to couple therapy complaining about their differing sexual needs. They each felt caught up in a cycle of events that they felt powerless to change. The end point of this cycle was that ultimately Beth felt she had to give in to Tom's insistent sexual demands. After about 18 sessions of therapy the couple came to realize that their behaviour around sex was for both of them a way of dealing with fears about rejection. They had both been raised in situations where they often felt very insecure, the result of Beth's parents separating when she was 3, and of Tom's father dying when he was 11. They had each developed an unconscious need for someone to help them contain their anxieties in relation to earlier separation and loss. As the end of therapy approached, despite having previously made progress, both Beth and Tom became more argumentative with each other in the session. They became unable to agree on anything, alternately sneering at the other and falling silent for long periods of time.

The therapist felt an overwhelming sense that she had failed, and with four sessions to go she was beginning to think that it had all been a waste of time. During supervision she herself became argumentative, leading the supervisor to wonder whether these reactions were in any sense associated with the impending loss of therapy that this couple was going to experience. The therapist wanted to offer more, and yet felt constrained by the time limit. It was suggested that she drew on her countertransference reaction in the remaining work with the couple. As a result the last three sessions dealt with the feeling of fear, anxiety, loss and anger that Beth and Tom had about their past and current experiences, including worries about failing each other and the therapist.

The example of Tom and Beth shows how powerful feelings of loss surrounding past and current experience need to be acknowledged openly and worked through. This is especially the case when there have been changes in sexual function and in other aspects of the relationship, such as through illness, separation, death or ageing. Such events can seriously test couples' ability to cope. This happens particularly where lack of good and secure internal objects leaves individuals with little resistance against the experience of feeling undermined, and prevents them adapting to change and loss. In women this can often be clearly seen in the consequences following on from children leaving home and the menopause. The corollary for men includes changes in employment in later years, and a decline in their ability to function sexually during this stage of life. The public interest in the debate surrounding Viagra and its availability shows the importance people attach to continuing to function sexually. For some clients the loss of full sexual functioning can provoke a serious loss of confidence, which in turn may lead to depression.

Brennan, aged 50, described his current relationship in terms of periods of adequate sexual functioning followed by times when he lost his erections and in response withdrew emotionally and physically. He had been married twice before, and both marriages were childless. In both instances his partners left him without warning. The second marriage was unsuccessful sexually, and during this time he started to lose interest in sex. He described the current relationship as happy and committed, and his only worry was his erectile problem. Following a discussion about whether he needed to come on his own to therapy, or with his partner, he decided to attend alone, which he did for about thirty sessions.

During Brennan's therapy his erection difficulties were formulated as a symptom of more widespread difficulties. His inability to keep his erection was symbolic of his struggle to hold on to both his longing for intimacy, and his fear of a close relationship. The periods of sexual inadequacy had generated a profound loss of confidence and a tendency towards self-denigration. However, the sexual symptoms allowed him to withdraw emotionally and so controlled the level of closeness in the relationship. During these periods of anxiety he felt overwhelmed and depressed, needing to be alone and wanting to avoid sex. His reluctance to involve his partner in therapy was interpreted as an extension of his difficulties with intimacy. In the course of therapy the therapist looked with him at two conflicting sides to him: his need for intimacy, and his need to cut himself off from people.

As therapy progressed he became more depressed and despairing, and had to take sick leave from work for a month. This was interpreted as his way of expressing anxieties and conflicts about his growing dependency in the therapeutic relationship. He was worried that he would become so depressed that he could not carry on his normal life, and in fact he did withdraw from most of his usual activities. He also revealed his despairing feelings about himself, his sense of failure and his underlying ambivalence towards his parents. His fragile internal object world was configured around an idealized, distant father and an over-critical but exciting mother. His sexual and relationship struggles embodied this split, whereby periods of excitement were followed by periods of distance. His sexual arousal difficulties occurred when he could no longer contain both aspects because the conflict between them had become too great. He regained his sexual potency when he was able to cope with his ambivalence and integrate these conflicting feelings, rather than direct the negative aspects of them against himself.

Working psychodynamically with sexual problems

A key part of working psychodynamically with sexual problems is an awareness of the defences identified in the formulation of an individual's or a couple's problem (see Table 5.9). The understanding of defences may need to be modified as the work progresses, but they provide a focus for making appropriate interventions. For example, looking first at women with *impaired sexual interest*, some have a narcissistic partner who is focused on his own needs, not just sexually but also more generally. The extent to which this can be worked with depends on the degree of this narcissism. At the extreme no progress is possible without the partner having individual therapy, but the nature of his defences often means that such a person does not see any need to change. In other instances it is more possible to facilitate change, such as when the man can appreciate that by meeting more of his partner's needs his needs will also be satisfied. Some men are able to work towards becoming more empathic and taking into account the partner's needs, especially when as part of the work they can obtain reassurance that their own needs are considered important.

In a relationship where the woman uses projection or projective identification to deal with negative aspects of herself, sex may be avoided in order to maintain distance from these unwanted and projected parts of herself. For example, where his aggression is being projected, the woman may say she is not interested in sexual contact because her partner is being so attacking. In most instances projections go both ways between partners. These need to be addressed by helping each partner to withdraw and work with their own projections, which may or may not be directly connected to sexual issues. This process depends on helping clients to recognize what is happening in the couple relationship, and being prepared to own and work on their part of the process.

> Chantel and Stuart had been married for 13 years, and had two children. They described their marriage as stormy, with difficulties that had started during their first year together. However, up to two years ago their sex life had been enjoyable for both of them, and one of the few areas about which they both could agree. Since Chantel had lost her interest in sex their general relationship had deteriorated, and they were both extremely frustrated and argumentative. They attended for therapy over a period of a year, and were able to identify how their mutual and conscious attraction to each other was based on wanting to marry a successful good-looking partner. Chantel saw Stuart as ambitious and able to cope with anything life threw at him, while Stuart saw Chantel as someone who was dependable and thoughtful about others.

They both felt that the other had qualities that they themselves initially desired, but these same qualities now formed part of their complaints about each other. Chantel felt that Stuart spent more time at work than with her, while Stuart complained that Chantel was more interested in the children than him. An interpretation was offered that sought to identify how their mutual projections worked to protect them from aspects of themselves, in particular how much they needed each other, but how this seemed to be denied, or channelled into other areas of their lives such as children and work. Chantel's loss of libido seemed to have upset this balance and she had withdrawn increasingly from her need for a physical relationship with Stuart by going to bed earlier and avoiding opportunities for sex. She was angry with Stuart for wanting to have this aspect of their relationship, yet it seemed prior to this she had enjoyed sex. Stuart for his part had found it difficult to think about their difficulties, and had up to a few years ago projected his fears and needs for intimacy into Chantel, identifying her as the needy one rather than himself.

This balance had been upset recently since they began to experience sexual difficulties. The beginning of Chantel's difficulties had coincided with her 10-year-old daughter starting menstruation. This had provoked many feelings for her, including a memory of her own menses, which had been difficult for her. It seemed that this event was associated with loss of control and Chantel's abiding fear of being overwhelmed. Her marriage to Stuart had brought relief from these feelings as he was always in control, and she had unconsciously projected her need to be in control into Stuart. This couple's relationship was based on defending themselves from fears of loss of control and intimacy by the use of projection.

Dissociation may be employed as a defence, particularly when sexual feelings arouse anxiety. For example difficulties in integrating the idea of a self as a sexual woman with the role of mother can lead to a dissociation from the former resulting in a loss of interest in sex. Sometimes this conflict is experienced consciously when women have recently given birth and their bodies and emotions are constantly moving between the maternal and the sexual. For instance, breast feeding the baby and then allowing the breast to be sexual with a partner can provoke discomfort in some women. Another origin of dissociation may be an experience of sexual abuse as children who are abused in this way often use dissociation to cope with what is happening to them. This can then establish a pattern of response to sexual contact which leads some women to dissociate in the same way during sexual activity as an adult. Others who have been abused or uncared for as children regress when they come into a relationship with an understanding partner, as this person comes to take on the role of replacement father towards whom sexual feelings are experienced as inappropriate. Problems of *lack of arousal* can involve similar processes of dissociation and may also result from repression.

Orgasmic dysfunction can be related to schizoid fears where the 'letting go' involved in orgasm is threatening because it raises anxieties about loss of self. Similarly negative feelings produced by the associations with sexual contact can trigger the denial or repression of sexual arousal, and makes achieving orgasm difficult. Laboratory studies have shown that some women can produce the physiological response of orgasm, but report no subjective experience of it. This may show these defences at work.

Vaginismus is a form of somatization, whereby split-off feelings and thoughts that are difficult to allow into consciousness are expressed in a physical symptom. For example, a relationship problem may be split off and dealt with in this way. *Dyspareunia* usually has a physical cause, although it is not unusual for it to be caused by a combination of organic and emotional problems. Sometimes enabling the client to obtain localized medication for such conditions as thrush or vaginitis to give symptomatic relief allows the therapist and client to address the psychological aspects of client's problems in a more effective way. Inasmuch as the cause is psychological, it can be dealt with psychodynamically as a form of somatization, as shown in the example of Josephine.

> Josephine, who had dyspareunia, also had regular bouts of vaginal thrush that had been treated with creams and pessaries, but the symptoms were alleviated only to return a few months later. Josephine described feeling bad about herself, and how this resulted in her avoiding sex with her partner. She started to feel that sex was dirty and that in some way the thrush was symbolizing this. Her therapy lasted about six months and the main focus was helping her to deal with difficulties about her body and sexuality.

In particular she worked through her feelings towards her vagina, which seemed to be a container for her bad feelings about sex and her negative introjects about her femaleness.

The various *sexual phobias* can be seen as projections of anxieties on to a particular activity as a way of avoiding an even greater anxiety. A phobia of touching male genitals may cover anxieties about being active rather than passive sexually. The meaning ascribed to being a sexual woman can invoke difficult feelings for some women, and avoiding sex or sexual arousal enables the woman to defend herself psychically from this conflict. For some women this situation can be temporarily reversed when they are engaging in sex in order to conceive, as such activity is briefly turned from a bad into a good object. Others seek alternative ways of conceiving, usually some form of artificial insemination using their partner's semen.

Turning to male problems, *erectile dysfunction* can involve a number of defences. Identification with a partner may raise anxieties about homosexuality associated with the penetration involved in sexual intercourse. Unconscious fears of being overwhelmed may result in erectile dysfunction, preventing intercourse and keeping the man differentiated from his partner. It commonly represents an attempt to regulate intimacy, with penetration representing a threat to autonomy. Alternatively, it may reflect a difficulty related to sexual object choice, as when a man is trying to deny homosexual attraction. In some instances it can also be a form of somatization, with similar roots to vaginismus in women, where unexpressed feelings are avoided and acted out. Genital pain with no clear physical cause may or may not be associated with erection problems, and it can usefully be treated as somatization, although the possibility of an undiscovered physical cause must also be kept in mind.

Both erectile dysfunction and *premature ejaculation* can be related to idealization: to fears about defiling the partner, or to sex with the man's partner being experienced as inappropriate or anxiety provoking, because such activity is not compatible with the idealized image of the partner. This is particularly so where the idealization has a maternal content. Premature ejaculation can be an expression of hostility towards the woman or to women generally, by depriving the partner of pleasure and satisfaction. Projection can result in impaired sexual interest, retarded and non-ejaculation and sexual phobias of various kinds. In each case the need to avoid the projected objects leads to a problem that in effect decreases intimate sexual contact. *Retarded and non-ejaculation* can result from the attempt to deny sexual feelings as well as an expression of ambivalence towards the partner, or women more generally. *Lack of sexual interest* is sometimes found in men who use intellectualization as a general defence against emotional experiences, especially experiences involving powerful and potentially uncontrollable feelings. *Genital pain* can have a physical cause, but where this cannot be established it may be a form of somatization.

> Peter, aged 33, presented with collapsing erections and an inability to have intercourse. His problems started after he tried to have intercourse with his current girlfriend. Despite finding her supportive he was now unable to maintain an erection sufficient for penetrative sex. Two years ago his partner of ten years left him with no explanation or warning. Following on from this he had gone through a protracted divorce, during which he had to borrow a substantial amount of money to buy his ex-wife's share of the marital home. He maintained that this had been difficult at the time, but claimed that this part of his life was now over and that he had made a new start. Moreover he said that he felt no hostility towards his previous partner and had just accepted what had happened. Clearly many of the problem issues resulting from the breakdown of the marriage and its aftermath had been repressed or denied, and had emerged in a new relationship as these insecurities were aroused.

Looking at sexual problems emerging primarily in the relationship, *differences of interest in sex* can result from a conflict between the need to merge and to differentiate, or from projections and splitting. *Difficulties in communicating about sex* can result either from over-differentiation or from over-identification between partners. *A general relationship difficulty causing a sexual problem* can often be helpfully seen in some instances as a somatic projection of the general problem, and in others as a reflection of shared emotional immaturity.

> Sheena and Tobias had been married for 25 years and had two grown-up daughters who no longer lived at home. They were married when they were both 18, when she

was pregnant with their first child. Tobias had experienced intermittent erection difficulties for the past three years, but during the last year intercourse had happened only twice. Sheena was very distressed at the interview, and described how she felt upset with him. In addition to being upset by the sexual problem, she felt Tobias had no time for her. In particular he was continually late home from work and when he was at home was always pre-occupied with work. She had tried to organize a holiday, but he would not commit himself to any dates. Tobias felt Sheena was being unreasonable, as his work was what provided for them.

During the first interview Sheena and Tobias could agree on nothing, including how long Tobias had been experiencing his difficulties. Their hostility towards each other was very clear. It was suggested that perhaps Tobias's sexual difficulty was symptomatic of more widespread difficulties that they were experiencing with each other. It seemed as if they had differing expectations of each other, but that communicating these and finding a compromise that suited them both was difficult. There always seemed to have to be a winner and a loser in their arguments, which it appeared served the function of helping them to feel differentiated from each other.

Processes in working psychodynamically with sexual problems

A psychodynamic approach to sexual problems involves the same processes that are used with other kinds of problem. *Interpreta-*

Table 6.1 Processes within psychodynamic counselling and psychotherapy

- interpretation
- insight
- working through
- resistance
- clarification
- confrontation
- transference
- acting out
- countertransference

tions are offered that facilitate *insight* and to enable problems to be *worked through* and *resistances* overcome. These include interventions aiding *clarification* and appropriate *confrontation*. Interpretations are also framed in response to the client's *transference* and *acting out* and the counsellor's *countertransference*.

The term *interpretation* has been used in a number of different ways, including the unconscious meaning and significance of the material brought by clients, the communication of these inferences and *all* comments made by the therapist. Rather than enter a semantic debate, it is perhaps better to describe specific kinds of intervention that can be of value in working with sexual problems. Some interventions may be specifically aimed at bringing about change through the medium of insight. An example of this may be pointing out the apparent similarity of a woman's partner to her father. The term 'content interpretation' is used to refer to the translation of surface material into deeper meaning, usually with reference to childhood material. So, the counsellor may suggest that perhaps someone's aversion to being approached sexually in a certain way has its roots in her childhood sexual abuse. Symbolic interpretations are suggestions of symbolic meanings as they appear in dreams, slips of the tongue, and so on.

The aim of a defence interpretation is to show the client the mechanisms and manoeuvres he or she uses to deal with the painful thoughts and feelings around an issue. Suggestions may also be made about their origin. Transference interpretations are concerned with the here-and-now of the relationship in the consulting room. These have a particular role in aiding the withdrawal of projections from a partner. There has been much discussion of the relationship between therapeutic progress and the making of correct interpretations. Glover (1955) suggests that inexact, inaccurate and incomplete interpretations may still result in therapeutic progress by the provision of an alternative system of organization for the client. In fact it can be rather unnerving for the client if the therapist is always right!

The type of *insight* that is of value to clients needs to extend beyond intellectual knowledge about their sexual difficulties. The kind of insight needed is that which either releases some emotion surrounding the difficulties or their causes, or involves some other aspect of a feeling state. However, intellectual insight can sometimes be valuable in containing problems. For example, the realization of a connection between childhood sexual abuse and lack of interest in sex may be accompanied by anger, or sadness, or both. There may also be a sense of relief when some understanding of the problem has been gained, especially when it has up to this point been surrounded with mystery. Insight also helps facilitate the creation of an understanding and observing ego. The process of insight into sexual problems may involve such areas as the effect of early experiences, the reasons behind partner choice, the function of symptoms, and the projections that are being put onto a partner. It is important to distinguish insight from the idea of a cure of the problem, as insight alone does not necessarily lead to therapeutic change. Clients are often disappointed when an increased understanding of the psychological reasons for their sexual problem does not immediately produce change.

> Tariq attended the sex therapy clinic because he was concerned about his promiscuous behaviour, which involved picking men up in local toilets for sex. He was married with two children, but his partner was unaware of his sexual activities outside their relationship. Tariq had no desire to leave the relationship, and maintained that he loved his wife, but at the same time felt that his sexual needs could not be fully met within their relationship. During sex with his partner he fantasized about his sexual interactions with the men he met. One insight he gained in therapy was the realization that his attachment needs were met within the marriage, but his sexual needs were largely split off and contained in this other hidden part of his life.

Working through makes insight more effective by addressing the resistances which keep insight into the sexual difficulty from leading to change. It can often involve going over the same ground again and again, a process which to some clients can feel like going round in circles. 'Sessions in this phase can feel plodding, laborious, repetitive, and uninspired. Resolution comes piecemeal, until one day it looks as though the work is almost done' (Scharff and Scharff 1991: 121). However, it is not realistic to think that unconscious impulses, conflicts, fantasies and defences can be worked through in any linear, organized way. The main tools available to the psychodynamic therapist and counsellor to help in working through are *interpretation, clarification, confrontation*, and working with the *transference* and *countertransference*. Balint warns against over-focusing on the negative, as the harmony and satisfaction are often more difficult for the outsider to see than the disharmony and dissatisfaction, but if one takes a closer look they can be found to be present even in the most unexpected places. We have found, in our therapeutic work with marriages under tension, that hidden loyalties and satisfactions are our most valuable allies.

(Balint 1993: 43)

A good concise definition of working through is the one offered by Klein:

Freud has postulated the process of *working through* as an essential part of the psychoanalytic procedure. To put it in a nutshell, this means enabling the patient to experience his emotions, anxieties, and past situations over and over again both in relation to the analyst and to different people and situations in the patient's present and past life.

(Klein 1959: 255)

There are elements and forces within clients which oppose the treatment process. It is important to understand the reasons for such *resistance*. One reason for resistance is where the counselling threatens to undo adaptations made by the client. An example of this is resistance against the recovery of a repressed memory of a traumatic sexual event. There will be additional resistance where the past is revived in a more vivid way in therapy, such as where the transference involves reactions to a person who abused the client. Commonly there are secondary gains from symptoms, and it is not surprising that some resolutions may be resisted. A sexual problem may enable the avoidance of intimacy or give excuse for an affair. There may be resistance because of the client's sense of guilt or their need for punishment. This may be particularly relevant in working towards an enjoyable sexual relationship. Changes brought about by the therapy may lead to real difficulties in the client's relationship with important persons whom they might not want to face. For example, a sexual problem can be a defence against the recognition that the relationship as a whole is not viable. In such an instance the resolution of the sexual difficulty may be resisted because the person does not want the relationship to end or because of the difficulties that might arise if it was consummated, as in the example of Gary.

Gary, aged 30, presented with an absence of erections. He was an insulin-dependent diabetic who had spent the last 12 years since his diagnosis trying as far as possible to ignore his condition. His GP suggested that his lack of erections was probably due to nerve and vascular damage arising from this condition. At the assessment Gary talked openly about his neglect of himself and how he had worried that he would end up with an erectile problem, although this still had not motivated him to act differently. He also spoke of how his father had died a year ago of a heart attack and how difficult life without him had been. Despite an absence of erections during sex and in the early morning Gary could achieve an erection for masturbation. This he estimated to be about half as good as that of which he used to be capable. He agreed that perhaps there was some unresolved psychological difficulties for him currently and in particular he had very ambivalent feelings about his current relationship. This was shown most clearly by the fact that he was having a relationship with his best friend's wife. Gary saw their marital problems as unconnected to him, as they had existed prior to his involvement, and rationalized the situation by stating that they had not been able to have sexual intercourse. His sexual problem prevented him from taking the relationship further and his rationalizations defended him from the guilt that he felt about his behaviour.

Sometimes therapy involves a threat to a client's self-esteem, which is particularly so when shame is activated. Working with sexual material is likely to put many clients in touch with such feelings. Resistance can also be prompted by the threat of the implications of a cure, and the loss of the counsellor that this will entail. Working through involves the clients giving up adaptive solutions to certain situations which they have habitually used. However, such solutions take time to unlearn, so resistance can operate while such unlearning is taking place. Finally, it is important to be aware that resistance can arise from clumsy, inappropriate or unhelpful interventions, such as introducing culturally specific ideas and values to clients with whom they are inappropriate.

Clarification is needed when the therapy has become unfocused or diffuse, or where the client has become lost in the details of the material. In addressing a sexual problem it is easy for sessions to open up a large range of couple and individual issues. It is important to clarify with clients in such situations why this might be happening and whether the work needs to be refocused on the original problem. It is also valuable to elucidate any material particularly related to the sexual problem and to separate this out from the more extraneous material. The aim of *confrontation* is to enable the client to recognize something which has been avoided, with the aim of working on it more explicitly. In working with couples it is particularly important to recognize that there may be a powerful collusion in their relationship to avoid certain matters. The overall purpose is to overcome resistance to change. As such, it is important that confrontation does not take place too early, or at a point where it cannot be received. The danger is that rather than overcoming resistance, a premature or inappropriate confrontation merely engenders even stronger resistance around the material.

Greenson gives a useful reminder of core nature of *transference* as

> the experiencing of feelings, drives, attitudes, fantasies and defences towards a person in the present which do not befit that person but are a repetition of reactions originating in regard to significant persons of early childhood, unconsciously displaced onto figures in the present. The two outstanding characteristics of a transference reaction are: it is a representation and it is inappropriate.
>
> (Greenson 1967: 155)

Thus the female counsellor may be experienced as the mother who disapproved of sex, so that the same inhibitions are awakened in the counselling session as belonged originally to the relationship with the mother. One aspect of transference of which a counsellor needs to be particularly aware is the unconscious (often subtle) attempt to manipulate and provoke situations with others that are repetitions of earlier experiences and relationships. Thus a client who experienced his mother as disapproving of sex may try to provoke disapproval of his sexuality from the counsellor, who clearly needs to be vigilant to this possibility. An important part of the work with clients is to contain and deal with *acting out*, both in the sense of the sessions bringing material to the surface which is enacted rather than remembered, and habitual, defensive ways of acting. Bateman and Holmes (1995: 195) say that acting out 'implies a regression to a prereflective, pre-verbal level, a belief in the magical effect of action, and a desperate need to get a response from the external world'.

The important task for counsellors and therapists is to try to contain all forms of acting out. Sexual acting out can be particularly hazardous, leading in some cases to unwanted pregnancies, HIV or sexual abuse.

> Keiran, aged 26, asked for help because of his inability to stop using prostitutes. He was apparently happily married, and his partner of two years had no idea about this. During therapy it became clear that his wife Stephanie represented safe, boring and predictable sex, whereas the visits to the prostitutes were exciting and risky. However, the majority of the time he felt emotionally deflated and very guilty after sex with a prostitute. At this point it was no longer exciting, and he returned home feeling awful, resolving not to behave in this way again. Despite this, his behaviour continued and he was eventually arrested for kerb crawling. Keiran managed to keep his secret life from his wife until he was arrested for drink driving in the local red light district and the police returned him home without a car. It was suggested to Kieran that his behaviour reflected a split within his emotional world between the exciting risk-taking part and the security-seeking part. He could not allow both these parts together into his sexual relating, fearing the consequences of doing so.

Sometimes the involvement of other professionals leads to difficulties in helping clients contain their behaviour. In particular, such a third party can offer the opportunity for acting out unresolved Oedipal issues, as the following case study illustrates.

> David came to the clinic with excessive concerns about the size of his penis. He was anxiously and compulsively pre-occupied with checking his penis throughout the day. After three appointments the therapist was contacted by David's GP, who expressed concerns about David's state of mind. The following week David came for his appointment, and the therapist mentioned the GP's telephone call. David admitted that he was anxious and that he was finding therapy difficult, but he expressed a need to come, and said that he was finding it useful. Therapy progressed slowly, and David used the time to discuss his lack of sexual experience, his poor self-image, and his fears that therapy would confirm his fears of inadequacy. Three months into

therapy a letter was sent by the GP to the consultant in the clinic expressing lack of confidence in the therapist dealing with the case. The GP said that he was no longer able to fund the therapy after a consultation with his patient that morning, where David had expressed serious doubts at the effectiveness of the help being offered. The therapist was surprised at this letter as David had not mentioned any such concerns to him. It transpired that David had been visiting his GP two or three times per week while he was in therapy and had been discussing suicidal thoughts. The client had successfully sabotaged his therapy by acting out his split-off destructive feelings away from the therapy session, projecting his own feelings of inadequacy onto the therapist via the GP.

Countertransference is often used in a general sense to describe the totality of the therapist's feelings and attitudes towards the client. Originally countertransference was seen purely in a negative sense, as something that gets in the way, but a major positive development took place with the recognition of countertransference as a potential aid in helping to understand the hidden meaning of material brought. One way in which this is done is by therapists recognizing feeling and thoughts in themselves that might have been projected by the client. The counsellor may become aware of rising emotionally tinged reactions to the client which cannot immediately be linked to surface content, but indicate the existence of something which is being forced onto the counsellor. For example, a man bringing an erectile problem to counselling may seem calm and talk very calmly about it, while the counsellor experiences an anxiety that she does not recognize as belonging to her. This may be a clue to the client's true emotional reaction to the problem. The counsellor's or therapist's awareness of his or her own responses can in this way provide an additional avenue into an individual's or couple's unconscious thoughts and feelings.

Sexual material picked up from clients in this way clearly has the potential to provoke unhelpful responses in a therapist if it activates his or her own inner conflicts. These can disturb both the understanding of what is going on in the therapy and how it is conducted, for example where resistance in the therapist leads to blind spots in relation to client material. Where working with a client evokes an important figure from childhood, the therapist is in danger of producing responses that belong at least partly to that relationship. If the therapist is unduly anxious about the therapy relationship, this is also likely to disturb the communication between therapist and client. For some practitioners their personal sexual history and current circumstances can lead to difficulties with some clients; for all practitioners there exist specific limitations which will be brought out by particular clients. All these possibilities highlight the need for counsellors to have good supervision as well as personal counselling or therapy if necessary. At one extreme there is always potential for sexual acting out with clients, with catastrophic consequences. But in all this, it is important not to lose sight of the appropriate or normal responses which the therapist has, which are important therapeutic allies as the basis for empathy and understanding.

Ethical issues

Working with psychosexual problems with couples and individuals involves particular pressures that arise from a conscious realization that intimate sexual and relationship practices are inextricably linked with personal morality and value systems. Alongside the usual need to work to high ethical standards, there are specific considerations that can arise when working with sexual aspects of clients' lives, which need careful attention. Many relate to the countertransference issues we have already discussed. Inevitably psychotherapists and counsellors bring their own beliefs and values to bear on their work, and it is important that therapists have a conscious awareness of how these assumptions about relationships and sexual practices affect their interpretations of the client's difficulties. Values that operate at conscious level (e.g. women should be treated as equals, sex is an important part of a relationship) are more easily addressed than those that exist at an unconscious level and are difficult to access. These common clinical issues and questions have been referred by Holmes (1996) as the 'ethical countertransference', and working with these forms part of maintaining an ethical practice where clients do not have the therapist's own values superimposed upon them. Supervision is one process through which therapists may become more aware of how these are operating – was I too interested in the male partner's sexual fantasies? Did I identify with the female partner too closely?

The idea of competencies in relation to sexual problems

makes it especially important that counsellors do not claim, or appear to imply, competence in areas of work for which they either have not been trained, or do not possess the capability. It is essential to be able to recognize and monitor limits to competence and to discuss this in supervision, as well as arranging consultations or referrals as needed.

Another ethical issue is the maintenance of proper boundaries when addressing sexual problems. It is particularly crucial, as many of the most destructive ethical breaches in therapy involve sexual contact within the therapeutic relationship. The nature of the material may result in sexualized or seductive transference feelings that need to be processed within supervision. Allowing the supervisee to acknowledge such processes enables such feelings to be deconstructed and opens up the possibility that these unconscious or conscious communications form part of the client's defensive system. Not abusing the counselling relationship sexually does not just mean keeping appropriate physical boundaries, but also refraining from actively sexualizing the transference, or attempting to elicit sexual material for the counsellor's own gratification. Respect for the client's autonomy involves allowing clients time to work round to disclosing sensitive or difficult sexual material and accepting that there may be some aspects about which they do not wish to talk.

Working with couples can present particular ethical tensions, in response to the importance of balancing the needs of the couple with those of one or both individuals. It is a real dilemma if certain material, such as the sexual abuse as a child of one of the couple, seems to require individual attention. The case for this can be very strong, although it might be quite disruptive to the couple work in progress. However, it may be useful to the couple if they can help identify what areas of difficulty one of them needs help with and to separate out these issues to enable the individual to seek additional help. For example, additional help is sometimes required if one of the individuals has a long-standing psychiatric condition; supporting individuals to seek out further help can enable the couple to concentrate on working together. It is important to recognize that with some sexual practices there are risks of infection or danger to the client, including legal and medical risks. Ultimately therapists have a responsibility to help the client acknowledge these aspects; the therapist may need to set limits on the kind of help that can be offered. This was the case with a man in his forties who came for help because he could not stop exposing himself at work. Both he and his employers saw therapy as the solution to his difficulties, and wanted the therapist to acknowledge in writing that his attendance at these appointments would help him cease his behaviour. No assurance of this kind could be given, and the man ceased therapy after four appointments. Another kind of predicament arises from a consultation where an elderly couple presented for therapy, one of whom was showing signs of dementia. During the consultation the couple described their sexual practices, but it was unclear how much the dementing partner was able to enter consensually into sexual activity.

Every counsellor has a limit to the type of thoughts and actions that he or she can contend with in working with clients. There can be internal or external pressures to work with anything that might be presented by clients, but this should be resisted. A distinction needs to be made between problem reactions and sexual prejudices that need to be worked through, and valid personal, ethical and religious positions. Some counsellors do not feel able to work with perpetrators of sexual abuse. This applies particularly to those who work extensively with sexual abuse victims, and those who themselves have been sexually abused. For some religious groups certain sexual practices are unacceptable, and counsellors who are adherents of such faiths should not have their beliefs pathologized and be forced to choose between them and their profession.

Psychodynamic supervision and personal therapy

Supervision of psychodynamic work with sexual problems needs to cover three main areas: monitoring the therapeutic process, dealing with countertransference issues and the maintenance of appropriate boundaries. Supervisors of psychodynamic psychosexual work need to be able to help the supervisee integrate the physical and psychological aspects of the presenting problem to prevent further splitting of the difficulty. Working within the limits of the therapist's competence may necessitate asking for medical, psychiatric opinion or further investigations, but this does not mean that the counsellor cannot integrate this within a psychodynamic frame.

Jay was referred to the psychosexual clinic with dyspareunia. She had suffered from this for ten years but had only just admitted the problem to her partner and her GP. It became apparent that Jay was very passive sexually, and often had intercourse without being sufficiently aroused. Her passivity was reflected in many areas of her relationship with her partner, whom she allowed to dominate in all the decisions that affected them. During the course of therapy Jay began to work through these difficulties and spoke of the similar kinds of problem she had experienced with her sister. Therapy progressed over a period of six months and focused on Jay's need to defend herself against her demanding, needy self which she projected into her partner.

Her difficulties with pain continued despite significant changes taking place in her relationship, where she began to take more control. It was suggested to the therapist in supervision that Jay needed an internal examination to exclude any persistent organic difficulties associated with certain skin disorders or infections. With Jay's permission a nurse member of staff within the clinic saw her, and laboratory tests revealed a persistent chlamydia infection that had caused an area of inflammation, which in certain sexual positions would become more irritated. This intervention and its consequences were explored within therapy and integrated and understood as part of the overall picture of Jay's difficulties. Within supervision it was also necessary to discuss the parallel process between Jay's deferential attitude to her partner and the therapist's feeling that she had no choice but to go along with the supervisor's recommendation about physical investigation. This allowed supervision to continue in a safe and containing way, without feelings and thoughts being split off, denied or ignored.

In monitoring the therapeutic process it is important for the supervisee to be helped in maintaining an appropriate balance between focus on the sexual problem and more general explorations. Over-focusing on the sexual difficulty may mean missing related areas that need to be worked through, but there can also be a risk that the core of the work becomes lost in a mass of individual or couple material. Narrative information is important, but supervisees working psychodynamically need help to identify the process aspects of therapy, and to help them access their countertransference. Through this, supervisees can be helped to extend their understanding of their clients' internal and unconscious struggles, and will be supported with their often difficult feelings that can arise in the context of working with such intimate areas of people's lives. Sometimes these reactions contain the supervisee's own personal material, and it is the responsibility of the supervisor to point out when this occurs and to suggest seeking personal therapy. Recognizing when this boundary is reached is part of the task of supervision.

Problems that need to be addressed in personal therapy are where strong reactions are judged to be more related to the counsellor's own unresolved personal material than to projections from clients. Personal therapy offers those working with sexual problems the opportunity to explore and resolve reactions to sexual material that are considered to be problem areas. It provides an arena where a counsellor can look at how these are provoked, as well as work through unresolved issues. Other worthwhile matters that can be addressed are the counsellor's own sexual and couple relationship experiences, and the effect of social and cultural influences.

The limits to competence form another area that can usefully be addressed in supervision. Such limits do not just involve knowing about psychodynamic therapy competences but also about medical, psychiatric and legal matters. Supervisors must ensure that such areas are not avoided but are brought up for discussion. In bringing such matters to supervisees' attention supervisors need to provide an appropriate balance of support and challenge in the discussion of the case material. This balance will be largely determined by how experienced the supervisee is in this area of work. It may be difficult for a supervisor to challenge experienced therapists, as they can feel threatened by this process of self-reflection, as though their practice is being questioned, and because of the tendency for 'colleague' collusions to develop. In particular, child protection issues continue to be an area provoking great anxiety among therapists, who are likely at some point to have clients whose behaviour towards children concerns them. In practice supervisors need to alert therapists to these issues, who may in turn need to raise these with clients. Ignoring or avoiding these concerns only perpetuates the problem. Helping clients to state how far they are actually behaving abusively, or thinking about it, is important in opening up this area for discussion, but does not in itself necessarily safeguard those at risk. The client will not generally be able to resolve the situation immediately and may not even stay in therapy to sort their difficulties out, as the example of Terry demonstrates.

Terry, aged 55, presented with erectile difficulties, of which he had become aware over the last 18 months. During the assessment he described his relationships with his partner and with his 23-year-old stepson. Terry said that he felt warm and affectionate to his stepson, but his son had ceased any contact with him a number of years back. We explored this further and he went on to describe loving this child and helping to prepare him for manhood. It sounded like sex had occurred between this man and his stepson, yet Terry never indicated this directly. It was suggested that he bring his partner to the follow-up assessment to explore further what was happening. This following interview was traumatic, as Terry's partner Rita described how her son had recently confided to her his sexual experiences with his stepfather. Terry refused to accept that he had done anything wrong, and for most of the interview insisted that he had not come to the appointment to discuss this matter. It was suggested that perhaps it could form part of the discussions, as it was difficult to ignore. Despite his agreement he did not attend any subsequent appointments. The therapist was left with a number of reactions to process, the most difficult being a sense of numbness that seemed illustrative of Terry's reaction to the fact that he had abused his stepchild, but tried to rationalize it away.

Psychodynamic supervision of psychosexual work is an integral component in a therapist's ability to work with the conscious and unconscious aspects of presenting sexual problems. Working with couples can provoke additional pressures on the therapist's ability to keep the focus of the work on the couple and their unconscious partnership in their difficulties. It is not uncommon in supervision that therapists need to look closely at how they either become aligned with one party or the other. Such problems in processing the psychodynamic work of couples have been discussed by Haldane and Vincent (1998). In some instances therapists may lose their observing self because of the complexities of the interactions involved in couples work. This can be caused by the restimulation of Oedipal issues for all those in the room, which can result in the therapist feeling overwhelmed, attacked or excluded, and 'as a result the capacity to think and reflect is lost' (Haldane and Vincent 1998: 391). The challenge for therapists who work with couples is to attempt to identify with their supervisor the defensive strategies that both couples and therapists use to ward off anxiety, instead of facing up to or confronting these issues.

Other areas that may be explored include emotional reactions to hearing about certain sexual practices, and situations that raise questions of values and ethics. The maintenance of proper boundaries when addressing sexual problems is particularly crucial, as many of the most destructive ethical breaches in therapy involve sexual contact within the therapeutic relationship. Supervisors need to help counsellors recognize when the transference becomes over-sexualized or too seductive and how to respond appropriately. It is also important to address ethical aspects as they arise within supervision.

Conclusion

Physical expressions of sexuality are mediated through a person's inner object relations as a necessary and vital part both of maintaining couple relationships and individual well-being. As such, many other approaches to sexual problems on their own cannot provide a comprehensive approach. While mechanical and pharmacological treatments have extended treatment options, it is not sufficient that sexual problems are seen as just technical or hydraulic difficulties. Similarly, theories focusing on behavioural and cognitive aspects on their own have shortcomings, with the result that sometimes other approaches are combined with these. An example of this is Crowe and Ridley's (1990) behavioural-systems approach to couple relationship and sexual difficulties. There has been less attention given to theoretical ideas surrounding the use of psychodynamic concepts alongside behavioural ones in addressing sexual problems, although the general idea of combining these theories is not new (Daines 1992).

One reason for the tendency to marginalize psychodynamic therapy of sexual problems is that research into psychodynamic approaches to sexual problems has been rare. This itself is partly a result of the dominance of other approaches within sex therapy over the last thirty years, but it is also a result of psychodynamic practitioners' lack of interest in research. Certainly within sex therapy the historical influences of medicine and behaviour therapy have skewed research towards quantitative rather than qualitative outcomes. Within psychodynamic sex therapy the goal of an absence of sexual symptomology is one quantitative measure that might be used to assess the successful outcome of psychotherapy. However, other measures, such as the quality of people's subjective experience of themselves and their relationships, are vital, but more difficult to measure.

Understanding and applying the kind of psychodynamic approaches to sexual problems we have described enables practitioners to offer clients an opportunity to resolve their sexual problems and explore their sexuality in an enriching way. Clients gain valuable insights and discover and work through aspects of themselves and their relationships that have caused difficulty. This process is difficult to structure and can sometimes be complex and confusing, as people come in contact with, and work with, unconscious aspects of their sexuality and relationships. What starts out, though, as an uncertain journey can end up as a route to lasting change.

Appendix 1

Further reading

Britton, R., Feldham, M. and O'Shaughnessy, E. (1989) *The Oedipus Complex Today: Clinical Implications*. London: Karnac.

Freud, Sigmund (1905) Three essays on the theory of sexuality, in Sigmund Freud (edited J. Strachey and A. Richards) *The Penguin Freud Library Vol. 7, On Sexuality*. Harmondsworth: Penguin, pp. 33–155.

Kaplan, H. (1974) *The New Sex Therapy*. New York: Brunner/Mazel.

Pincus, L. and Dare, C. (1978) *Secrets in the Family*. London: Faber.

Scharff, D.E. (1982) *The Sexual Relationship*. London: Routledge.

Scharff, D.E. and Scharff, J.S. (1991) *Object Relations Couple Therapy*. Northvale, NJ: Jason Aronson.

Appendix 2

Glossary

N.b. many psychodynamic terms are used with different meanings by different writers. The definitions below apply to usage in this book and aim to reflect their most common usage in psychodynamic counselling theory.

acting out dealing with internal conflicts by repeating a pattern from the past. This is often used in the context of it being provoked by the content of counselling or therapy.

cardiovascular disease disease of the heart and/or blood vessels.

clarification the process of separation of significant from extraneous material, thus bringing it into focus and clarifying detail.

confrontation the process of drawing the client's attention to particular things and making them explicit, with the aim that the client recognizes what is being avoided and needs further exploration.

countertransference the counsellor's responses and reactions to the client.

depressive position Klein uses this term to describe the stage at which the child realizes that his love and hate are directed towards the same object: the mother. There is an associated experience of ambivalence and the need to make reparation for the damage that the hate is imagined to have caused.

dyspareunia pain experienced by a woman during sexual intercourse.

episiotomy a cut made in a woman's perineum to facilitate childbirth.

erectile dysfunction difficulty in obtaining and/or maintaining an erection.

fantasy ideas relating to imagined objects (cf. phantasy – ideas relating to internalized objects).

genito-urinary referring to the genitals and urinary tract.

identification the process by which a person extends identity into another, for example to avoid responsibility or vicariously enjoy the other's activities.

impaired sexual interest reduction in, or lack of, sexual interest.

insight realization that involves emotional release as well as intellectual aspects.

internalization the process by which objects in the outside world are changed into images that then form part of our mental schema.

interpretation interventions by the counsellor that convey inferences and conclusions about the meaning and significance of the client's communication and behaviour.

introjection the process by which an external object is replaced by an internal imagined object.

masochism the obtaining of erotic pleasure from the inflicting of pain by another.

narcissism a tendency to use the self as the point of reference around which experience is organized.

non-ejaculation an inability to ejaculate (cf. retarded ejaculation).

object-relations theory the theory based on a person's relationship with internal and external objects, in contrast to the drive theory of Freud. Developed by Klein, Fairbairn and Winnicott.

orgasmic dysfunction in women, a difficulty in having, or inability to have, an orgasm.

phantasy ideas relating to internalized objects (cf. fantasy – ideas relating to imagined objects).

premature ejaculation an inability to delay ejaculation.

primary sexual problem a sexual problem that has always existed in sexual relationships with another.

projection the process by which parts of the self are imagined to be located outside of oneself.

projective identification the process by which a person relates to the self or parts of the self by locating them in another person.

psychoanalytic relating to the body of theory initially developed by Freud and developed by other psychoanalysts.

psychodynamic relating to the body of knowledge based on a division of the mind between the conscious and the unconscious.

psychogenic psychological in origin.

regression a re-experiencing of earlier stages of personality development.

reparative a defence process designed to reduce guilt towards an object about which the person feels ambivalent.

retarded ejaculation difficulty in ejaculation leading to sexual dissatisfaction.

resistance the aspects within the client that oppose the counselling process.

sadism the obtaining of erotic pleasure by inflicting pain on another.

schizoid the use of defences, particularly splitting, to deal with guilt and depression.

secondary sexual problem A sexual problem that has not always existed in sexual relationships with another.

sexual phobias undue anxiety produced by sexual situations or contact, leading to their avoidance.

transference the projection by clients onto their counsellor or psycho-therapist of attitudes, feelings, ideas and reactions that belong to previous important figures in the client's life.

vaginismus painful spasm in the muscle of the vagina leading to pain on and/or difficulty with, penetration.

vascular relating to blood vessels.

working through the process by which resistances that prevent change are overcome.

Appendix 3

Useful addresses

British Association for Counselling
1 Regent Place, Rugby, Warwickshire CV21 2PJ
01788 578328

British Association for Sexual and Relationship Therapy
P.O. Box 13686, London SW20 9ZH
0181 543 2707

Counselling in Primary Care Trust
First floor, Majestic House, High Street, Staines TW18 4DG
01784 441782

UK Council for Psychotherapy
167–9 Portland Street, London W1N 5NB
0171 436 3002

References

Abraham, K. (1924) A short study of the development of the libido, viewed in the light of mental disorders, in K. Abraham (1979) *Selected Papers*. London: Maresfield, pp. 418–50.

Althof, S.E. and Turner, L.A. (1992) Self-injection therapy and external vacuum devices in the treatment of erectile disfunction: methods and outcome, in R.C. Rosen and S.R. Leiblum (eds) *Erectile Disorders, Assessment and Treatment*. New York: Guilford Press, pp. 283–309.

Althof, S.E., Turner, L.A., Levine, S.B., Risen, C., Kursch, G., Bodner, D. and Resnick, M. (1991) Long term use of self-injection therapy of papaverine and phentolamine, *Journal of Sex and Marital Therapy*, 17: 101–12.

Baggaley, M.R., Hirst, J.F. and Watson, J.P. (1996) Outcome of patients referred to a psychosexual clinic with erectile failure, *Sexual and Marital Therapy*, 11: 123–30.

Balfour, F. and Richards, J. (1995) History of the British Confederation of Psychotherapists, *British Journal of Psychotherapy*, 11: 422–6.

Balint, E. (1993) Unconscious communications between husband and wife, in S. Ruszczynski (ed.) *Psychotherapy with Couples*. London: Karnac.

Bancroft, J. (1989) *Human Sexuality and its Problems*. London: Churchill Livingstone.

Bancroft, J. (1997) Sexual problems, in D.M. Clark and C.G. Fairburn (eds) *The Science and Practice of Cognitive Behaviour Therapy*. Oxford: Oxford University Press, pp. 243–57.

Barsanti, M. (1997) 'On Lacan, "Mirror" and "Phallus"', unpublished paper.

Bateman, A. and Holmes, J. (1995) *Introduction to Psychoanalysis. Contemporary Theory and Practice*. London: Routledge.

164 *Psychodynamic approaches to sexual problems*

Belliveau, F. and Richter, L.R. (1971) *Understanding Human Sexual Inadequacy*. London: Hodder and Stoughton.

Black, J. (1988) Sexual dysfunction and dyspareunia in the otherwise normal pelvis, *Sexual and Marital Therapy*, 3: 213–21.

Bowen, M. (1972) Toward the differentiation of self in one's own family, in J.L. Framo (ed.) *Family Interaction: A Dialogue Between Family Researchers and Family Therapists*. New York: Springer, pp. 111–73.

Britton, R. (1992) The Oedipus situation and the depressive position, in R. Anderson (ed.) *Clinical Lectures on Klein and Bion*. London: Routledge, pp. 34–45.

Britton, R., Feldham, M. and O'Shaughnessy, E. (1989) *The Oedipus Complex Today: Clinical Implications*. London: Karnac.

Bubenzer, D.L. and West, J.D. (1993) *Counselling Couples*. London: Sage.

Burnap, D.W. and Golden, J.S. (1967) Sexual problems in medical practice, *Journal of Medical Education*, 42: 673–80.

Campbell, T.W. (1995) Repressed memories and the statute of limitations: examining the data and weighing the consequences, *American Journal of Forensic Psychiatry*, 162: 25–45.

Clarkson, P. (1990) A multiplicity of psychotherapeutic relationships, *British Journal of Psychotherapy*, 7: 148–63.

Cleavely, E. (1993) Relationships: interaction, defences, and transformation, in S. Ruszczynski (ed.) *Psychotherapy with Couples*. London: Karnac, pp. 55–69.

Colman, W. (1993a) Marriage as a psychological container, in S. Ruszczynski (ed.) *Psychotherapy with Couples*. London: Karnac, pp. 70–96.

Colman, W. (1993b) The individual and the couple, in S. Ruszczynski (ed.) *Psychotherapy with Couples*. London: Karnac, pp. 126–41.

Crowe, M.J. (1985) Marital therapy – a behavioural-systems approach, in W. Dryden (ed.) *Marital Therapy in Britain*. London: Harper and Row, vol. 1, pp. 312–38.

Crowe, M. and Ridley, J. (1990) *Therapy with Couples*. London: Blackwell.

Daines, B. (1988) Assumptions and values in sexual and marital therapy, *Sexual and Marital Therapy*, 3: 149–64.

Daines, B. (1992) Behavioural-psychodynamic approaches to marital therapy – an exploration of possibilities, *Sexual and Marital Therapy*, 7: 65–77.

Daines, B., Gask, L. and Usherwood, T. (1997) *Medical and Psychiatric Issues in Counselling*. London: Sage.

Dallos, S. and Dallos, R. (1997) *Couples, Sex and Power: The Politics of Desire*. Buckingham: Open University Press.

Daniell, D. (1985) Marital therapy: the psychodynamic approach, in W. Dryden (ed.) *Marital Therapy in Britain*. London: Harper and Row, pp. 169–94.

D'Ardenne, P. and Mahtani, A. (1989) *Transcultural Counselling in Action*. London: Sage.

Dickinson, R.L. (1933) *Human Sex Anatomy*. Baltimore, MD: William and Wilkins.

Dickinson, R.L. and Pierson, H.H. (1925) The average sex life of the American woman, *Journal of the American Medical Association*, 85: 1113–17.

Dicks, H.V. (1967) *Marital Tensions*. London: RKP.

Draguns, J.G. (1981) The history, issues and current status of cross-cultural work, in A.J. Marsella and P.B. Pedersen (eds) *Cross-Cultural Counselling and Psychotherapy*. New York: Pergamon.

Edgcumbe, R. (1985) Modes of communication: the differentiation of somatic and verbal expression, *Psychoanalytic Study of the Child*, 39: 137–54.

Eichenbaum, C. and Orbach, S. (1985) *Understanding Women*. London: Penguin.

Ellis, H. (1929) *Man and Woman*. Boston, MA: Houghton Mifflin.

Ellis, H. (1936) *Studies in the Psychology of Sex*. New York: Random House.

Ellis, H. (1952) *Sex and Marriage*. New York: Random House.

Ellis, H. (1954) *Psychology of Sex* (2nd edition). New York: Emerson Books.

Ellis, M.L. (1987) Who speaks? Who listens? Different voices and different sexualities, *British Journal of Psychotherapy*, 13: 369–83.

Erikson, E.H. (1965) *Childhood and Society*. Harmondsworth: Penguin.

Fairbairn, W.R.D. (1954) *Psychoanalytic Studies of the Personality*. London: Routledge.

Fiedler, F.E. (1950) A comparison of therapeutic relationships in psychoanalytic, non-directive and Adlerian therapy, *Journal of Consulting Psychology*, 14: 121–53.

Fink, B. (1997) *A Clinical Introduction to Lacanian Psychoanalysis*. Cambridge, MA: Harvard University Press.

Fisher, J. (1993) The impenetrable other: ambivalence and the Oedipal conflict in work with couples, in S. Ruszczynski (ed.) *Psychotherapy with Couples*. London: Karnac, pp. 142–6.

Fogel, G.I. and Myers, W.A. (eds) (1991) *Perversions and Near-Perversions in Clinical Practice*. New Haven, CN: Yale University Press.

Foucault, M. (1984) *The History of Sexuality*. London: Peregrine Books.

Framo, J.L. (1965) Rationale and technique of intensive family therapy, in I. Boszormenyi-Nagy and J.L. Framo (eds) *Intensive Family Therapy: Theoretical and Practical Aspects*. New York: Harper and Row, pp. 143–212.

Framo, J.L. (1976) Family origin as a therapeutic resource for adults in marital and family therapy, *Family Process*, 15: 193–210.

Freud, Sigmund (edited J. Strachey and A. Richards) *The Penguin Freud Library*. Harmondsworth: Penguin (abbreviated PFL).

   vol. 2, *New Introductory Lectures on Psychoanalysis*.

   vol. 7, *On Sexuality*.

   vol. 8, *Case Histories I*.

Freud, Sigmund (1905) Three essays on the theory of sexuality, PFL (1977a), vol. 7, pp. 33–155.

Freud, Sigmund (1909) Analysis of a phobia in a five year old boy, PFL (1977b), vol. 8, pp. 165–317.

Freud, Sigmund (1910) Special type of object choice made by men, PFL (1977a), vol. 7, pp. 227–42.

Freud, Sigmund (1912) On the universal tendency to debasement in the sphere of love, PFL (1977a), vol. 7, pp. 243–60.

Freud, Sigmund (1925) Some psychical consequences of the anatomical distinction between the sexes, PFL (1977), vol. 7, pp. 323–44.

Freud, Sigmund (1933) PFL (1971), vol. 2.

Gardner, F. (1995) Being in the know: thoughts on training, prestige and knowledge, *British Journal of Psychotherapy*, 11: 427–35.

Glover, E. (1955) *The Technique of Psycho-Analysis*. New York: International Universities Press.

Godschalk, M., Gheorghiu, D., Chen, J., Katz, P.G. and Mulligan, T. (1996) Long-term efficacy of the new formulation of prostaglandin E1 as treatment for erectile dysfunction, *Journal of Urology*, 156: 80–1.

Graziottin, A. (1998) Organic and psychological factors in vulval pain: implications for management, *Sexual and Marital Therapy*, 13: 329–38.

Greenberg, J.R. and Mitchell, S.A. (1983) *Object Relations in Psychoanalytic Theory*. Cambridge, MA: Harvard University Press.

Greenson, R.R. (1967) *The Technique and Practice of Psychotherapy*. London: Hogarth Press.

Gudjonsson, G.H. (1986) Sexual variations: assessment and treatment in clinical practice, *Sexual and Marital Therapy*, 1: 191–214.

Guntrip, H. (1968) *Schizoid Phenomena, Object Relations and the Self*. London: Karnac.

Gustafson, J.P. (1986) *The Complex Secret of Brief Psychotherapy*. New York: Norton.

Haldane, D. and Vincent, C. (1998) Threesomes in psychodynamic couple therapy, *Sexual and Marital Therapy*, 13: 385–96.

Hardy, G.E., Barkham, M., Shapiro, D.A., Reynolds, S., Rees, A. and Stiles, W.B. (1995) Credibility and outcome of cognitive-behavioural and psychodynamic-interpersonal psychotherapy, *British Journal of Clinical Psychology*, 34: 555–69.

Hawton, K. (1985) *Sex Therapy: A Practical Guide*. Oxford: Oxford University Press.

Heine, R.W. (1953) A comparison of patients' reports on psychotherapeutic experience with psychoanalytic, nondirective and Alderian therapists, *American Journal of Psychotherapy*, 7: 16–23.

Hiller, J. (1993) Psychoanalytic concepts and psychosexual therapy: a suggested integration, *Sexual and Marital Therapy*, 8: 9–26.

Hiller, J. (1996) Female sexual arousal and its impairment: the psychodynamics of non-organic coital pain, *Sexual and Marital Therapy*, 11: 55–75.

Hirst, F.J. and Watson, P.J. (1997) Therapy for sexual and relationship problems: the effects on outcome of attending as an individual or as a couple, *Sexual and Marital Therapy*, 12: 321–37.

Holmes, J. (1996) Values in psychotherapy, *American Journal of Psychotherapy*, 50: 259–73.

Horrocks, R. (1997) *An Introduction to the Study of Sexuality*. London: Macmillan.

Horton, R. (1967) African traditional thought and Western science I and II, *Africa*, 37: 50–71 and 151–87.

Jacobs, M. (1994) Psychodynamic counselling: an identity achieved? *Psychodynamic Counselling*, 1: 79–92.

Jehu, D. (1979) *Sexual Dysfunction: A Behavioural Approach to Causation, Assessment and Treatment*. New York: Wiley.

Jones, R.F., Sullivan, M.J.L. and Ritvo, P.G. (1995) *Relationships in Chronic Illness and Disability*. London: Sage.

Jung, C.G. (1925) Marriage as a psychological relationship, *The Collected Works of C.G. Jung vol. 17* (1954). London: RKP, pp. 189–201.

Kaplan, H. (1974) *The New Sex Therapy*. New York: Brunner/Mazel.

Kaplan, H.S. (1977) *Disorders of Desire*. New York: Brunner/Mazel.

Kaplan, H. (1987) *Sexual Aversion, Sexual Phobias, and Panic Disorder*. New York: Brunner/Mazel.

Kayser, K. (1993) *When Love Dies: The Process of Marital Disaffection*. New York: Guilford Press.

Kinsey, A.C. *et al.* (1948) *Sexual Behaviour in the Human Male*. Philadelphia: W.B. Saunders.

Kinsey, A.C. *et al.* (1953) *Sexual Behaviour in the Human Female*. Philadelphia: W.B. Saunders.

Kitzinger, S. (1983) *Women's Experience of Sex*. Harmondsworth: Penguin.

Klein, M. (1959) Our adult world and its roots in infancy, in M. Klein (1997) *Envy and Gratitude and Other Works 1946–1963*. London: Vintage.

Lago, C. and Thompson, J. (1996) *Race, Culture and Counselling*. Buckingham: Open University Press.

Lavee, Y. (1991) Western and non-western human sexuality: implications for clinical practice, *Journal of Sex and Marital Therapy*, 17: 203–13.

Leader, D. and Groves, J. (1995) *Lacan for Beginners*. Cambridge: Icon.

Leiblum, S.R. and Rosen, R.C. (eds) (1992) *Erectile Disorders, Assessment and Treatment*. New York: Guilford Press.

Lemaire, A. (1977) *Jacques Lacan*. London: RKP.

Levin, S.B., Risen C.B. and Althof, A.E. (1990) Essay on the diagnosis and nature of paraphilia, *Journal of Sex and Marital Therapy*, 16: 89–102.

Levine, S.B. (1992) Intrapsychic and interpersonal aspects of impotence: psychogenic erectile dysfunction, in R.C. Rosen and S.R. Leiblum (eds) *Erectile Disorders, Assessment and Treatment*. New York: Guilford Press, pp. 255–82.

Lidmilla, A. (1996) What do we mean by psychodynamic? A contribution to the development of a model, *British Journal of Psychotherapy*, 12: 435–46.

LoPiccolo, J. (1992) Postmodern sex therapy for erectile failure, in R.C.

Rosen and S.R. Leiblum (eds) *Erectile Disorders, Assessment and Treatment*. New York: Guilford Press, pp. 171–97.

Lorion, R.P. and Parron, L.D. (1985) Countering the countertransference: a strategy for treating the untreatable, in P. Pederson (ed.) *Handbook of Crosscultural Counseling and Therapy*. Westport, CN: Greenwood Press.

Lyons, A. (1993) Husbands and wives: the mysterious choice, in S. Ruszczynski (ed.) *Psychotherapy with Couples*. London: Karnac, pp. 44–54.

Lyons, A. and Mattinson, J. (1993) Individuation in marriage, in S. Ruszczynski (ed.) *Psychotherapy with Couples*. London: Karnac, pp. 104–25.

Maguire, M. (1995) *Men, Women, Passion and Power*. London: Routledge.

Maguire, V. (1973) Counsellor effectiveness: a critical review, *British Journal of Guidance and Counselling*, 1: 38–50.

Malan, D.H. (1976) *The Frontiers of Brief Psychotherapy*. New York: Plenum.

Malan, D.H. (1979) *Individual Psychotherapy and the Science of Psychodynamics*. London: Butterworth.

Masters, W.H. and Johnson, V.E. (1966) *Human Sexual Response*. Boston, MA: Little, Brown and Co.

Masters, W.H. and Johnson, V.E. (1970) *Human Sexual Inadequacy*. Boston, MA: Little, Brown and Co.

McDougall, J. (1989) *Theatres of the Body*. London: Free Association Books.

McKay, M. (1988) Subsets of vulvodynia, *Journal of Reproductive Medicine*, 38: 9–13.

McLeod, J. (1998) *An Introduction to Counselling*. Buckingham: Open University Press.

Meissner, W.W. (1978) The conceptualization of marriage from a psychoanalytic perspective, in T.J. Paolino and B.S. McCrady (eds) *Marriage and Marital Therapy: Psychoanalytic, Behavioural and Systems Perspectives*. New York: Bruner/Mazel, pp. 25–88.

Meltzer, D. (1973) *Sexual States of Mind*. Ballinluig: Clunie Press.

Morrison, L.A. and Shapiro, D.A. (1987) Expectancy and outcome in prescriptive vs. exploratory psychotherapy, *British Journal of Clinical Psychology*, 26: 59–60.

Norcross, J.C. (1997) Light and shadow of the integrative process in psychotherapy, post-conference seminar reported in P. Clarkson, Beyond schoolism, *Counsellor and Psychotherapist Dialogue* (1998) 1: 13–19.

O'Brien, M. (1990) The place of men in a gender sensitive therapy, in R.J. Perelberg and A. Miller (eds) *Gender and Power in Families*. London: Routledge, pp. 170–240.

O'Connor, N. and Ryan, J. (1993) *Wild Desires and Mistaken Identities; Lesbianism and Psychoanalysis*. London: Virago.

Petrak, J. and Keane, F. (1998) Cultural beliefs and the treatment of sexual dysfunction: an overview, *Sexual Dysfunction*, 1: 13–17.

Pincus, L. (1976) *Death and the Family*. London: Faber.

Pincus, L. and Dare, C. (1978) *Secrets in the Family*. London: Faber.

Pokorny, M. (1995) History of the United Kingdom Council for Psychotherapy, *British Journal of Psychotherapy*, 11: 415–21.

Polonsky, D.C. and Nadelson, C.C. (1982) Marital discord and the wish for sex therapy, *Psychiatric Annals*, 12: 685–95.

Pop, H.G. and Hudson, I. (1995) Can memories of childhood sexual abuse be repressed? *Psychological Medicine*, 25: 121–6.

Power-Smith, P. (1984) 'Sex and the elderly', unpublished manuscript.

Power-Smith, P. (1992) Encounters with older lesbians in psychiatric practice, *Sexual and Marital Therapy*, 7: 79–86.

Ransom, D.C. (1980) Love, love problems, and family therapy, in K.S. Pope (ed.) *On Love and Loving: Psychological Perspectives on the Nature and Experience of Romantic Love*. San Francisco: Jossey Bass, pp. 244–65.

Reece, R. (1988) Special issues in the etiologies and treatments of sexual problems among gay men, *Journal of Homosexuality*, 15: 43–57.

Riley, A.J. (1998) Integrated approaches to therapy, *Sexual and Marital Therapy*, 13: 229–31.

Roberts, R.E.I. (1996) Forensic gynaecology and sexual assault, in J.W.W. Studd (ed.) *The Yearbook of the Royal College of Obstetricians and Gynaecologists*. London: RCOG Press, pp. 70–88.

Rokke, P.D., Carter, A.S., Rehm, L.P. and Veltum, L.G. (1990) Comparative credibility of current treatments for depression, *Psychotherapy*, 27: 235–42.

Rosen, G.M. (1987) Self-help treatment books and the commercialization of psychotherapy, *American Psychologist*, 42: 46–51.

Rosen, I. (1987) The psychoanalytical approach (Symposium on sexual dysfunction), *British Journal of Psychiatry*, 140: 85–93.

Rust, J., Golombok, S. and Pickard, S. (1987) Marital problems in general practice, *Sexual and Marital Therapy*, 2: 127–30.

Rycroft, C. (1972) *A Critical Dictionary of Psychoanalysis*. Harmondsworth: Penguin.

Sandford, C.E. (1983) *Enjoy Sex in the Middle Years*. London: Martin Dunitz.

Sandford, C. and Beardsley, W. (1986) *Making Relationships Work*. London: Sheldon Press.

Schachter, J. (1997) The body of thought: psychoanalytic considerations on the mind–body relationship, *Psychoanalytic Psychotherapy*, 11: 211–19.

Scharff, D.E. (1982) *The Sexual Relationship*. London: Routledge.

Scharff, D.E. (1988) An object relations approach to inhibited desire, in S.R. Leiblum and R.C. Rosen, *Sexual Desire Disorders*. New York: Guilford Press, pp. 44–73.

Scharff, D.E. and Scharff, J.S. (1991) *Object Relations Couple Therapy*. Northvale, NJ: Jason Aronson.

Schover, L.R. and LoPiccolo, J. (1982) Treatment effectiveness for disorders of sexual desire, *Journal of Sexual and Marital Therapy*, 8: 179–97.

Segraves, R.T. (1982) *Marital Therapy: A Combined Psychodynamic-Behavioural Approach*. New York: Plenum.

Segraves, R.T. and Segraves K.B. (1998) Pharmacology for sexual disorders, *Sexual and Marital Therapy*, 13: 302–3.

Shapiro, D.A. (1981) Comparative credibility of treatment rationales: three tests of expectancy theory, *British Journal of Clinical Psychology*, 28: 111–22.

Skynner, A.C.R. (1976) *One Flesh: Separate Persons*. London: Constable.

Strong, B., Devault, C. and Sayad Werner, B. (1996) *Core Concepts in Human Sexuality*. London: Mayfield.

Stuntz, R.C. (1988) Assessment of organic factors in sexual dysfunctions, in R.A. Brown and J.R. Field (eds) *Treatment of Sexual Problems in Individual and Couples Therapy*. Maryland: PMA, pp. 187–208.

Synder, D.K. and Berg, P. (1983) Predicating couples' response to brief directive therapy, *Journal of Sex and Marital Therapy*, 9: 114–20.

UKCP (1997) *Recovered Memories of Abuse: Notes for Practitioners 1997*. London: UKCP.

Van der Velde, T.H. (1930) *Ideal Marriage*. New York: Covici-Friede.

Vance, C. (ed.) (1984) *Pleasure and Danger: Exploring Female Sexuality*. London: RKP.

Wilden, A. (1968) Translator's introduction to J. Lacan, *Speech and Language in Psychoanalysis*. London: Johns Hopkins University Press.

Wile, D.B. (1993) *Couples Therapy: A Nontraditional Approach*. New York: Wiley.

Winnicott, D.W. (1953) Mind and its relation to the psyche-soma, *Through Paediatrics to Psychoanalysis*. London: Hogarth Press, pp. 243–54.

Winnicott, D.W. (ed.) (1965) *The Maturational Process and the Facilitating Environment*. London: Karnac.

World Health Organization (1992) *The Classification of Mental and Behavioural Disorders. (ICD-10)* Geneva, WHO.

Wylie, K., Hallam-Jones, R., Coan, A. and Harrington, C. (1999) A review of the psychophenomenological aspects of vulval pain, *Sexual and Marital Therapy*, 14: 151–64.

Young, R.M. (1996) 'Is "perversion" obsolete?', Chapter 4 of *Whatever Happened to Human Nature?* Published on the internet at http://www.shef.ac.uk/~psysc/human/chapter4.html

Zinner, J. and Shapiro, R. (1974) The family as a single psychic identity: implications for acting out in adolescence, *International Review of Psycho-Analysis*, 1: 179–86.

Index